CHOOSING
to CHANGE

CAROLE LEWIS

Regal

A Division of Gospel Light
Ventura, California, U.S.A.

Published by Regal Books
A Division of Gospel Light
Ventura, California, U.S.A.
Printed in the U.S.A.

Regal Books is a ministry of Gospel Light, an evangelical Christian publisher dedicated to serving the local church. We believe God's vision for Gospel Light is to provide church leaders with biblical, user-friendly materials that will help them evangelize, disciple and minister to children, youth and families.

It is our prayer that this Regal book will help you discover biblical truth for your own life and help you meet the needs of others. May God richly bless you.

For a free catalog of resources from Regal Books/Gospel Light, please call your Christian supplier or contact us at 1-800-4-GOSPEL or www.regalbooks.com.

Cover Design by Barbara LeVan Fisher
Interior Design by Robert Williams
Revised edition edited by Rose Decaen

Library of Congress Cataloging-in-Publication Data
(applied for)

1 2 3 4 5 6 7 8 9 10 11 12 13 14 15 / 09 08 07 06 05 04 03 02 01

Rights for publishing this book in other languages are contracted by Gospel Literature International (GLINT). GLINT also provides technical help for the adaptation, translation and publishing of Bible study resources and books in scores of languages worldwide. For further information, write to GLINT, P.O. Box 4060, Ontario, CA 91761-1003, U.S.A. You may also send e-mail to Glintint@aol.com, or visit the GLINT website at www.glint.org.

To my husband, Johnny,

whose servant heart keeps my life from unraveling,

whose sense of humor assures that my life is never dull,

whose love and support enable me to do what I do.

CONTENTS

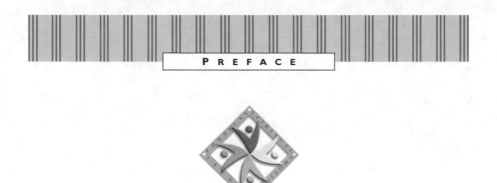
First Place is a program centered on Jesus Christ and His Lordship. The program is designed to bring balance into our lives in four areas: mental, physical, spiritual and emotional. When we realize that giving Christ first place is the answer to any hunger we might experience, we have assurance of complete healing for any need we face.

When I joined First Place in March of 1981, I had no idea of the changes that would take place in my life in the years ahead. I have learned that I have a choice in every change. Unless I choose to change, God will not be able to do the work that He desires in my life.

Oswald Chambers makes a statement about choices that I love: "Our choice is indelibly marked for time and eternity. What we decide makes our destiny, not what we have felt, nor what we have been moved to do, or inspired to see, but what we decide to do in a given crisis, it is that which makes or mars us."[1]

My prayer for you as you read this book is that you will be inspired and motivated to make the choices necessary for change to occur in your own life. God bless you in your journey of choices.

Note

1. Oswald Chambers, *The Best from All His Books*, vol. 2 (Nashville, TN: Oliver Nelson Books, 1989), p. 29.

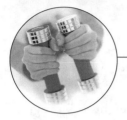
A STARTING PLACE:
THE FIRST PLACE
STORY

"For I know the plans I have for you," declares the LORD, "plans to prosper you and
not to harm you, plans to give you hope and a future. Then you will call upon me
and come and pray to me, and I will listen to you. You will seek me and find me when
you seek me with all your heart. I will be found by you," declares the LORD,
"and will bring you back from captivity."

JEREMIAH 29:11-14

I hadn't seen my friend Kay for some time, but both of us attended a baby shower in December of 1980. We'd grown up together and shared many wonderful experiences. She looked absolutely great. I said to her, "Kay, how could you do this to me?"

"Do what?"

"How could you lose weight and not tell me?"

"Carole, have you forgotten that we are going to be 40 next year? Do you want to be fat and 40?"

"Well, I really hadn't thought of it that way." Her honesty shocked me. I needed to lose about 20 pounds, the same 20 pounds I had repeatedly worked on for years. I began dieting when I was 13 years old. I tried practically every weight-loss plan available. My last approach had been a low-carbohydrate diet. Predictably, I lost the same 20 pounds I had lost before on every other plan. When I reached my goal, I thought I would never have that weight problem again. But I gained the pounds back. Seeing Kay reminded me of the cycle I was repeating. I thought, *Here I am again, with the same 20 pounds, and yes, I'm going to be 40 next year.*

When I read in our church paper that a new weight-loss program was starting in March of 1981, I became excited. I thought, *This is something that possibly will work for me.* The program was called First Place.

STEPPING OUT IN FAITH

First Place began at Houston's First Baptist Church with a group of 12 men and women. Each one felt that God intends for believers to be balanced in all areas of life—mental, physical, spiritual and emotional—and that God desires to help us in each area. This group met together and prayed that God would give a program to First Baptist that would meet the needs of the believers in that church. One of the 12 wrote the Bible study, another designed the cover, and another created all the forms that were used in the program.

When I attended the First Place orientation in March of 1981, I eagerly anticipated what God might want to do in my life. At that time, I didn't realize that God wanted to be Lord of my *entire* life. As a Christian I knew that God was sovereign. But I felt that He really wasn't interested in little things like my weight. I felt I should pray about bigger, more important things. Through my First Place group, God showed me that He has a sense of humor. He gave me a leader who didn't even have a weight problem! Sandy Griffin was the wife of the minister of activities and had been enlisted to lead the group because so many people had enrolled.

As I became acquainted with the First Place program, I came face-to-face with a spiritual problem that I had not confronted before: rebellion within me. Rebels don't think that rules are made for them, so I came into First Place picking and choosing what I was going to do. For example, I chose not to use the First Place Live-It food plan. I had recently lost 20 pounds—even though I had gained it back again—on a low-carbohydrate plan, and I thought I would just continue to follow the same plan.

Consequently, I came into First Place not eating a balanced diet. On this low-carbohydrate diet I didn't eat any bread or fruit. I ate four or five different vegetables and all the meat and fat I wanted as long as I consumed fewer than 1,200 calories a day.

I was losing weight, too. However, my Fact Sheet (which is now called a Commitment Record) would inevitably be returned with the question inscribed at the top, "Carole, what are you doing? This is not our food plan." Sandy knew I was following some other plan. Since she didn't have a weight problem herself, she had no idea what kind of plan I was following. Sandy never confronted me openly, so I never had to tell her why I wasn't following the First Place food plan.

As time went by, I lost the same 20 pounds. I was very pleased to have lost the weight. I loved the program. I loved the Bible study and the fellowship. But I had never followed the First Place food plan. Much to my surprise, Sandy recommended me to lead a group in the next session. She told Dottie Brewer, one of the founders of the program, that I had lost weight and Sandy thought I had leadership potential. That's how I became a First Place leader.

PUTTING GOD FIRST

In Jeremiah 29:11, God said, "I know the plans I have for you." God knew the plans He had for me back in March of 1981—plans for good and not for evil, plans to give me a future and a hope. As I began in earnest to lead First Place, I had a long way to go.

To begin with, I didn't even know what the Live-It plan was, so I set myself the task of learning it. In the early days of First Place, we used a book by Better Homes and Gardens called *Eat and Stay Slim*. I had to read the food section of that book several times even to begin to understand exchange eating. I did learn it and began to teach it to my group. What a joy I experienced leading that First Place group!

In January of 1981, the bottom suddenly dropped out of the Houston economy. Between the years of 1981 and 1985 many successful businesses and businessmen went broke. Thousands of families who had purchased homes at very high interest rates were forced to leave their homes to find work elsewhere. Many people were unable to sell their homes, so they were forced into foreclosure when they moved to other cities.

During this time, our family was undergoing some tremendous financial problems. My husband had his own business and struggled from 1982 to 1984 to keep it afloat. Finally in 1984, he had to give it up. I went to work in the education department at First Baptist Church in August of 1984 when my family was at a low point in our lives. In mid-December of 1984, God showed me that all our family had been going through was a means to draw me to Him—to give up my rebellious ways and let Him become Lord of everything about me.

I had no idea how to let God be Lord. How could I let go when I had been running my own life for so many years? A couple of weeks later, our pastor, Dr. John Bisagno, preached a sermon on the will of God. He said, "If you are here this morning and you know that God wants to change your will, you must know that He won't come in and work on your will without your permission to do so. If you will just pray this prayer this morning—'Lord, I'm not willing, but I'm willing to be made willing'— then that gives God permission to come in and work on your will."

That morning, as sincerely as I have ever prayed, I said, "Lord, that's where I am today. I am scared to death of what You might do if I give You control of every part of me. But my family is in such a terrible mess and I feel like I'm in such a mess spiritually and emotionally. I want to give You permission to work on my will." I'll never forget closing, "Please don't let it hurt too much." At that time I believed that if you were in the center of God's will, it had to be painful. I assumed you were sent to China or Africa; I certainly didn't want to go to either place! But I was willing to be willing. God began that very day to make the changes in my life that were necessary. The first change was choosing to let God work in the area of my will. Many choices were to come later, but this was the real starting point.

One of the first areas God chose to work on was the physical aspect of my life, so I began a walking program in October of 1984. Three months later I began a jogging program that I continued for 15 years until a knee injury brought me back to walking and bicycling for aerobic exercise. I have also added flexibility and strength training to my exercise program in the last few years. That's a change that I would never have dreamed possible when I started First Place. I had never been consistent with anything in my whole life. Everything I had attempted was a start-and-stop proposition. God wanted to see consistency in all the areas where I'd failed to follow through. God is so patient and loving. He just works on a little bit at a time. As we choose to allow Him to work in our lives, He always gets the job done no matter what it takes or how long. The idea that I have been exercising regularly for many years astounds me.

God also began to work in my life in the area of relationships. He knew I would be deeply involved with people, so He needed to make sure I really loved people the way He loved them. For years I had taught Sunday School and worked in the church, but I never had the love for people that God has. I felt that He knew how busy I was and that He understood that I didn't have the time to get involved in people's lives. I would teach them, but I never wanted to be a part of their pain.

In January of 1985, God began to change my heart toward my family, friends and coworkers. He began to show me the love He had for everybody I knew. He wanted me to demonstrate His kind of love. He tells us in Mark 12:30,31 how He wants us to love: "'Love the Lord your God with all your heart and with all your soul and with all your mind and with all your strength.' The second is this: 'Love your neighbor as yourself.'" To love my neighbor as myself—that's exactly where He began to work in my life.

SPREADING THE FIRST PLACE STORY

By 1983, other churches were beginning to ask for the First Place program. Those who had completed First Place and moved to other churches were asking, "How can we do First Place at our new church? This is too wonderful to give up." We had to make a decision. Dottie Brewer, the founder of the First Place program, presented First Place to a publisher in Dallas and proposed selling the program to them. They wanted to make it available to the public through Christian bookstores. However, on her way back to Houston, as Dottie was praying, she felt God really impressing her to keep the program at First Baptist Church and to train people to use it. She felt people would not know what to do with it if they purchased it in a bookstore. She also feared the buyer would not feel the need for the group support that we believe is so important in First Place.

Dottie decided we would keep the program in the church and let it grow at a slower pace. As people asked about First Place, we helped them get a program started. In 1986, we began to offer the program to churches. We still use the same format today. Representatives all over the United States teach leaders how to love people and care about them through leading a First Place group.

In 1985 and 1986, First Place didn't have a full-time staff person. Dottie Brewer was volunteering 20 to 30 hours a week. By July of 1987, First Place was being used in around 50 churches. At about this same time, the secretary who handled the First Place clerical duties was planning to take maternity leave. I was approached about taking over the First Place program.

Dottie was confident that I loved the program. She was also confident that my relationship with God had grown to the point where she felt she could step back and turn the program over to me. When I became the director of the First Place program, Dottie left me with some big shoes to fill. I will always admire her for the many ways she contributed to the launching of First Place.

Those first few months were hectic. I took all the orders over the phone and opened all the new accounts. I shipped a lot of the materials. I did the billing each month. I knew everyone who had an account with First Place and handled every facet of the work. In spite of my hectic schedule, it was a wonderful job. As the program grew, I was learning more and more about First Place. Little did I know the heartbreak that was to follow.

GRIEVING AND GROWING THROUGH CHANGE

God works in such miraculous ways. He knew when I went full-time with First Place in the summer of 1987 that Dottie was going to become ill in the fall of that same year. Her illness was very mysterious. She suffered from anemia for a year and the doctors treated her with iron. She had a tremendous amount of back pain. Although in pain, she continued with her regular activities, even skiing with her family in January of 1988. She went in and out of the hospital for tests. The doctors could not find the cause of her illness.

In July of 1988, Dottie was diagnosed with colon cancer and given three months to live. Dottie lived for eight months after the diagnosis. I spent many hours at Dottie's bedside, along with Kay Smith, who later became my associate. Little did we know how God was preparing us for the task ahead. Whenever Dottie wanted us with her at the hospital, we were there. God allowed us to see the depth of her spirituality. I sat with her at night and read her prayer journal. God showed me that she was a person who consistently prayed for those she loved and cared about.

God worked in my own heart during this time of pain and grief, watching Dottie's body deteriorate. Yet her heart was still strong because she had been an exercise walker for 15 years. It made me rethink my own exercise program: Did I want my body to outlive my heart? I realized that our days are in the Lord's hands, and none of us who know Him is going before the time He plans for us to come home. Until that time we need to be good stewards of our bodies, taking good care of our temples.

Dottie went home to be with the Lord on March 22, 1989. I'll never forget something she said about three weeks before she died. It was the last time she was in the hospital and though she was very sick, she never lost her sense of humor. Propped up on some pillows and knowing she wasn't going to live much longer, she said, "Carole, of all people, I would never have chosen you as director of First Place." We had a good laugh and talked about what a sense of humor God has.

BEGINNING YOUR JOURNEY: CHOOSING TO CHANGE

When He chooses us, we have a lot of decisions to make. And if we choose to follow Him, God can use even those of us who are rebels. He can take those of us who seemingly do not have anything to give Him and do great and mighty things with our lives. Each of us has a starting place. My starting place was certainly not glorious. But God was there. From the time we accept Jesus as our personal Savior, God promises never to leave us. We may attempt to control our own lives for years, but we have the assurance that the Holy Spirit is in our lives, working to mold us into the persons that God created us to be.

I'm so glad that you have a starting place where you can know that God is there in every choice that you will make. As you begin your journey in First Place, the things you see happen may not be monumental to you. But later on you will be able to say that God was there in the beginning. He's helped me make the choices that are going to change my life forever. I'm confident that He will do the same for you.

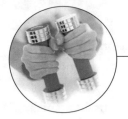
CHOOSING A LIFE OF BALANCE

Jesus grew in wisdom and stature, and in favor with God and men.

LUKE 2:52

The core of the First Place program is living a life of balance in all areas—mental, physical, spiritual and emotional. Balance is only possible in a life that has Jesus Christ at its center. After we become children of God, He continues to instill balance in our lives. Jesus Christ is our role model. He is the most balanced person who ever lived on this earth. I love the fact that He was as human as I am, yet without sin.

Let's look at the four areas of balance represented in the life of Christ, as illustrated in the passage of Scripture found in Luke 2:40-52:

And the child grew and became strong; he was filled with wisdom, and the grace of God was upon him.

Every year his parents went to Jerusalem for the Feast of the Passover. When he was twelve years old, they went up to the Feast, according to the custom. After the Feast was over, while his parents were returning home, the boy Jesus stayed behind in Jerusalem, but they were unaware of it. Thinking he was in their company, they traveled on for a day. Then they began looking for him among their relatives and friends. When they did not find him, they went back to Jerusalem to look for him. After three days they found him in the temple courts, sitting among the teachers, listening to them and asking them questions. Everyone who heard him was amazed at his understanding and his answers. When his parents saw him, they were astonished. His mother said to him, "Son, why have you treated us like this? Your father and I have been anxiously searching for you."

"Why were you searching for me?" he asked. "Didn't you know I had to be in my Father's house?" But they did not understand what he was saying to them.

Then he went down to Nazareth with them and was obedient to them. But his mother treasured all these things in her heart. And Jesus grew in wisdom and stature, and in favor with God and men.

MENTAL

When I think about Jesus having to grow mentally, I am filled with hope. Although Jesus was only 12 years old, the Temple scholars and teachers were astonished at what He had to say. Imagine what God could do with our minds if we obediently allowed Him to fill them with those things that are of true importance. In First Place, you are going to learn how to let God be the Lord of your mind, as well as your heart. You are going to learn how to fill your mind with Scripture as you listen to the Scripture memory audiocassettes/CDs in the car and while you exercise. As you recite a verse from memory each week when you get on the scale to weigh in, you will begin to form a lifelong habit that will literally change every part of your life.

You will also learn that the term "garbage in, garbage out" has great significance in the life of a Christian. For many years, I didn't realize that I was filling my mind with things that were of no eternal significance. In the early 1980s, my mom took my sister and me on a church-sponsored trip to Austria. It was a once-in-a-lifetime opportunity for us, and I was so excited about getting to go. In the airport, our minister of music was reading a book called *The Thornbirds*, and he encouraged me to buy a copy to read on the trip. I purchased a copy in the airport and began to read. During the bus tours through the beautiful Austrian countryside, my mom would urge me to look at something out the window of the bus. I would look up for a minute and then go right back to the book. When *The Thornbirds* was made into a miniseries on television a short time later, I had to laugh. I didn't even remember the story line. And I had missed a trip to Austria to read that book!

God doesn't pry our fingers open and take away from us those things that we think are so important. He gently begins to replace those things with ones of greater significance. Through this process we begin to see that He has a better plan for our lives.

In Houston we have a lot of "dead time" in freeway traffic. In 1985, I realized the need to fill the dead time. I decided this would be a wonderful time to fill my mind with the things of God. Audiocassettes would be the perfect solution. I felt the need not only for Scripture cassettes but also for motivational cassettes; however, they were a luxury I felt I could not afford. I mentioned this need in my First Place meeting. The very next week, a lady in my class arrived with a grocery sack full of cassettes. She said, "I want you to have these. My husband and I have been to every seminar that has ever come to town. These cassettes are all by motivational speakers. I don't need them back. Listen to them and then give them to others." I followed her advice and have loaned those cassettes to many people over the years.

As you identify your own dead time and allow God to fill it with thoughts that will enable you to grow, you will find yourself changing mentally, physically, spiritually and emotionally. God will begin to impress upon you the importance of filling your mind with what you need in order to be used to enrich the lives of other people. This process will be gradual, but mentally you will begin to find balance in your life that you've never had before.

Today, First Place has its own Scripture memory audiocassettes and CDs to help members memorize Scripture. The memory verses for each of the eight studies are on separate CDs and are included in the inside back cover of each Bible study. As you memorize Scripture, you will notice how God will begin to change you, through knowing His Word and applying it to your life.

PHYSICAL

Jesus grew not only in wisdom but also in stature. The pictures of Jesus that I remember from my childhood showed Him to be rather frail. However, the Jesus of the Scriptures is quite a different person. We know that Jesus was a carpenter by trade. Until He began his public ministry at age 30, He earned His living as a carpenter. He had to carry large pieces of wood and stone to build structures. His trade would have required great physical strength. We also know from Scripture that Jesus walked from Sidon to Tyre, which would have been a 40-mile trip, in one day (see Matt. 15:21-29). Instead of comfortable tennis shoes, He wore handmade sandals as He walked over rough and rugged terrain. Imagine some of the disciples following along, griping all the way. I would have complained also, had I been there.

We know also that Jesus carried His cross. It must have been very heavy and Jesus must have been strong and fit. When we say that we want to be like Jesus, do we really mean that? Do we want to take the best possible care of these bodies that God has given us so that we can live as long as possible to serve Him every day? Jesus, who was not lazy in any respect, calls us to follow His example.

One of the changes that you will encounter as you begin the First Place program will be learning to eat in a different way. When I started First Place, I wondered when I could quit doing the program and start eating what I wanted. That was my mind-set with each weight-loss program I tried. That's why I was always destined to gain back the weight I lost. I never thought of it as a lifestyle change.

Like me, many of you have never considered changing your lifestyle. Only with a lifestyle change was I able to quit the constant yo-yoing back and forth. With the First Place Live-It food program, you will be able to stabilize your weight.

You are also going to be asked to start an exercise program that will last the rest of your life. Some who enter First Place can just barely walk. Well, dear Christian, if that's all you can do today, then we're asking you to just barely walk. God will bless your efforts and He'll help you. Before you know it, you'll be walking three miles a day—or whatever goal you set for yourself. If you will give what you have to God, He'll multiply it and give it back to you in a way that you would never have believed possible. So be prepared for the many physical changes that will take place in your life.

SPIRITUAL

We know that Jesus grew not only in wisdom and in stature but also in favor with God. We know that Jesus was with God when God created the universe. He became God in flesh when He came to Earth to be born as a baby in Bethlehem. We know that He was sent here to be the Savior for our sin. During the brief time Jesus lived on Earth, why would He need to spend so much time with the Father? We are reminded throughout Scripture that Jesus got up early to pray. Apparently, Jesus felt time alone with His Father was a priority. That's why He had the confidence to say, "I do nothing on my own but speak just what the Father has taught me" (John 8:28).

When I began First Place, I believed that God had given me common sense and He expected me to use it! I knew His Word and I knew what to do. I acted impulsively many times and made decisions based on my own way of thinking. God has made tremendous changes in that area of my life. He's taught me to wait on Him. Following His lead, I've been able to make decisions based on His will, not my own. But I've had to be patient. I've had to be willing to wait, because God works in His time.

I believe there are areas in which all of us have trust problems with God. He's taught me to trust Him. When I teach a Sunday School class, I've learned to go before God and wait for His guidance. I continue to read and study through the week, but I've learned to depend on Him for the final outline. He always comes through. He always does more than I could ever ask when I trust Him.

If you are strong willed like me, God has to begin to show you that His way is best. Only by waiting on Him will you receive His best. He's proved Himself to me in so many ways in these years that I never want to walk out ahead of Him. We need to allow Him to make these changes.

We are not going to see them overnight. For God to make these changes, we have to make the right choices. We will have to choose to read His Word and to spend time in prayer. As we make those choices, He says that He'll manifest Himself to us—and He will. As I meet people at First Place conferences all over the country, I ask, "How much weight have you lost?" Many times I will hear a testimony such as this: "Well, I've lost 80 pounds in First Place. But that's not the most important benefit. I've had a life-changing spiritual experience." I know that will happen in your life, too. It's exciting to see what God's going to do as you begin to give Him first place in your life.

EMOTIONAL

Jesus not only grew in wisdom and in stature and in favor with God, but He also grew in favor with man. Just being around Jesus had a life-changing effect on people.

Jesus was walking through town and He spied Zacchaeus up in a tree. He said, "Zacchaeus, come down immediately. I must stay at your house today" (Luke 19:5). Zacchaeus scampered down and took Jesus home with him. His whole life was changed that day. God wants each of us to be changed by our relationship with Jesus. He wants others to be able to see Jesus by the way we live. Witnessing through our lifestyle may require us to experience change in the way we deal with our emotions.

Jesus was balanced emotionally. He was able to express His emotions, whether anger at the money changers, sadness at the death of Lazarus or joy at the wedding feast at Cana. He always expressed His feelings appropriately. He was in control of His emotions, not controlled by them.

Many of us live totally out of our emotions. We eat because of our emotional state. Whether we're happy, sad, depressed or anxious, it's a cause to eat. We eat as a way to celebrate important occasions. Eating becomes a way to deal with our emotions. We've been told that at least 80 percent of obese men and women have suffered some form of abuse, whether physical, mental, emotional or sexual. In our First Place program,

we have offered special First Place classes as an opportunity for partici-
pants to experience emotional healing. These classes last two hours, one
hour for the regular First Place meeting and one hour for sharing.

God is committed to our emotional healing from the moment we
accept Jesus. Those of us who suffer emotional pain must stay very close
to the side of God through daily prayer and Bible study. Only by retrain-
ing our emotions are we going to find wholeness. Only through God's
Word will that wholeness come to us. God promises to bless His Word.
If you have suffered abuse of any kind, your only hope is found in God
and in His Word. Trust Him to heal your life and make you a whole person by bringing emotional balance to your life.

As you memorize Scripture and also learn how to pray Scripture
back to God, you will begin to experience emotional healing. Each of the
First Place Bible studies will help you start your journey toward wholeness. We know that some of the most wonderful changes that will take
place in your life are going to be the changes in the emotional area.

In March of 1991, God showed me a Scripture confirming how He
sends emotional healing to His people. Isaiah 42:6,7 tells us:

> I, the LORD, have called you in righteousness; I will take hold of
> your hand. I will keep you and will make you to be a covenant for
> the people and a light for the Gentiles, to open eyes that are
> blind, to free captives from prison and to release from the dun-
> geon those who sit in darkness.

In June of 1992, I attended a MasterLife dinner, at which Avery Willis
gave a testimony about how the Life Support courses had started:
Claude King, T. W. Hunt and Avery were at a prayer retreat in the fall of
1990 when God gave them a Scripture. Avery began to quote the passage
from Isaiah that talked about bringing the prisoners out of their prison
and opening blind eyes. I was overcome with emotion. God had given me
the same Scripture only a year before. God confirms to His people what
He's going to do.

As you begin First Place, perhaps your life—as mine did—will mirror
Paul's description in Romans 7:15: "I do not understand what I do. For

what I want to do I do not do, but what I hate I do." But have hope. You can do all things in Christ Jesus.

It is my prayer that someday you will identify more with Romans 8:5,6:

> Those who live according to the sinful nature have their minds set on what that nature desires; but those who live in accordance with the Spirit have their minds set on what the Spirit desires. The mind of sinful man is death, but the mind controlled by the Spirit is life and peace.

You can expect life and peace as you choose balance in the mental, physical, spiritual and emotional areas of your life.

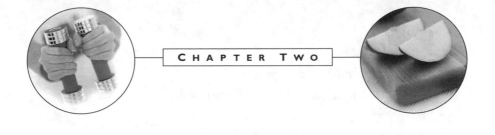

THE NINE COMMITMENTS OF FIRST PLACE

The First Place program consists of nine commitments that will help you draw closer to the Lord and aid you in establishing a solid and consistent Christian life. Each commitment is a necessary and important part of the goal of First Place: to become healthier and stronger in four areas of your life—mental, physical, spiritual and emotional. In short, First Place should lead you toward becoming the person God created you to be.

These commitments are written with the expectation that group members are Christians. We invite anyone into our program; however, if you are not a Christian, you will want to discuss your participation in the program with your group leader. The aim of First Place is a totally balanced Christian life, based on salvation through Jesus Christ. The name "First Place" is derived from the commitment to give Christ first place in your life (see Matt. 6:33). We invite you now to read Choosing Christ on pages 87-89.

Now let's take a look at the commitments themselves. Although they are not listed in order of priority, each element is essential in order for First Place to transform your life into a life of balance.

Commitment One:
Attendance—Choosing to Show Up
Faithful attendance at your weekly group meeting is essential.

Commitment Two:
Encouragement—Choosing to Reach Out to Others
Weekly, contact by phone, note or e-mail one person from your group.

Commitment Three:
Prayer—Choosing to Pray
Set aside time each day to be alone with the Lord in prayer.

Commitment Four:
Bible Reading—Choosing to Read God's Word
Read and study God's Word for direction in your life.

Commitment Five:
Scripture Memory Verse—Choosing to Memorize God's Word
Memorize one verse of Scripture every week.

Commitment Six:
Bible Study—Choosing to Study the Bible
Each week's Bible study is divided into daily assignments.

Commitment Seven:
Live-It Plan—Choosing to Eat Right
A food exchange plan helps you eat good balanced meals.

Commitment Eight:
Commitment Record—Choosing to be Accountable
This daily record helps you track your progress in the program.

Commitment Nine:
Exercise—Choosing to Exercise
Begin or continue an exercise program to insure physical fitness.

Now that you have been introduced to the First Place program commitments, perhaps you're thinking that they sound helpful, but you wonder if you can keep them. Let His Word assure you: "I can do everything through him who gives me strength" (Phil. 4:13).

In the pages that follow, the commitments will be explained in greater detail. You will see how and why they work. You will be inspired by the way lives have been changed through First Place and its commitments. You will see that choosing to change might well be the best decision you'll ever make.

CHOOSING TO SHOW UP

Where two or three come together in my name, there am I with them.

MATTHEW 18:20

Attendance is the first commitment of the First Place program. Group sessions for support and encouragement have been an important element of First Place since the program began, and we feel the communal experience is a key to the success of First Place.

Attending First Place meetings must be a priority in your life. If you're not there, you miss the bonding of the group. You miss what God did in the lives of group members during that particular meeting. You miss the support and the encouragement that the leader in the group will give you.

In the First Place program, attendance is so important that if you're not able to come to a group session, we ask you to call your leader or someone else in the group and let him or her know. Then the group can pray for you and the needs in your life. The commitment of group members to each other contributes to the realization that we are not alone in our struggle for health and wholeness. Others are cheering us on. We in turn cheer for them.

BONDING

The experience of one of our First Baptist Houston groups is a good example of the importance of bonding. Janice Campbell, one of our leaders, felt God leading her to start a First Place group for women who weighed more than 200 pounds. Janice had lost 130 pounds herself on

First Place. She felt God wanted her to reach out to these women, many of whom felt hopeless about losing weight.

During the orientation sessions for the next round of classes, Janice put an asterisk on the commitment form filled out by women in this weight category. Then she called them individually and asked them if they would be interested in such a group. Every one of them was very excited about participating.

However, at that first group meeting Janice had never seen so much hopelessness. These women had a long way to go and a lot of weight to lose. They were skeptical about their prospects for success. Janice began to question the wisdom of her idea. Yet after only the first week, the group began to bond together. Janice saw results as pounds were lost and spirits were lifted. After a few weeks, one of the ladies in the group asked, "After we weigh under 200 pounds, does that mean we have to leave this group?"

Fortunately, the answer was no. The group stayed together, supporting and encouraging one another. Their positive experience in group sessions represents the type of bonding that occurs in a First Place group.

However, bonding is possible only if group members show up. If you're not there, then people can't reach out to you in love. They can't put their arms around you; they can't assure you that they have had the same feelings or been in the same circumstances. The bonding aspect of First Place is one of the most important reasons for you to show up each week.

ENCOURAGEMENT

A little boy was always afraid when the light was turned out at night. His father assured him that Jesus was there with him. One night the father finished the bedtime story, and the little boy said his prayers. As the daddy walked out of the room, he turned out the light. In a minute, the little boy called him back into the room. The boy said, "Daddy, I know I shouldn't be afraid. I know that Jesus is here with me. But you know, sometimes I just need somebody with skin on."

People in your First Place group feel much the same way. They need that human contact and support—they need to know someone is there for them. I hear from groups all across our country that express the excitement members feel about the group experience. One such testimony came from Letha Mahan, who led a First Place group in Mountain Home, Arkansas:

> We began this great adventure with two groups that included 26 very committed members. . . . We laughed, wept, jumped for joy, screamed with frustration, increased our strength, learned our weaknesses and came to know each other to an immeasurable degree. The prayers that were answered can only be said to be miraculous.

ACCOUNTABILITY

Various reasons may tempt you to skip a group session. You may have had a bad week and eaten foods that you shouldn't have eaten. Maybe you know you didn't lose any weight, or possibly you gained some. Your inclination is not to attend that week, thinking that you will do better next week. We all have difficulty when we must face up to our weaknesses.

What usually happens, though, is that next week is even worse. Without the group's encouragement and with your own feelings of defeat to weigh you down, you may not want to go again the following week. After two or three weeks like this, you may want to drop out entirely. You'll try to justify leaving by saying "This just isn't a good time for me." Perhaps you think this scenario I've pictured is exaggerated. Unfortunately, I've seen this series of events happen time after time when members make the decision to stay away from their groups.

Someone once said 80 percent of life is showing up. I've found that to be very true in my own life. I have to show up for every one of the First Place commitments. For example, I have to show up to exercise. I can't remember a morning when I awoke and proclaimed, "Oh, this is wonderful. I get to exercise today." I'd rather stay home, drink coffee and read the paper. But exercise is a discipline that God has shown me is necessary in my life. So I get up, put on my clothes and show up for exercise. Many mornings I tell myself that I'm only going to walk a mile. I justify my actions by thinking, *At least I'm doing something that 95 percent of the world doesn't do. I'm showing up.* But God meets me at my point of obedience. As I begin my morning walk, someone will show up to walk with me. We share about what the Lord is doing in our lives and, invariably, I'll finish my walk and, most of the time, have walked farther than I had planned.

If I don't choose to show up, I won't exercise. The same principle applies to First Place group meetings. Refusal to show up for First Place meetings will not make your day any better. It could, in fact, make it worse. Therefore, we make the choice to show up.

As you begin or continue your First Place commitments, plan to make attendance at group sessions a priority in your life. Think it through when you are tempted to let minor distractions keep you away. Recognize that your success in the First Place program depends on each small step of obedience and self-discipline. You will find your self-esteem will grow as you make right choices in every area of your life.

CHOOSING TO REACH OUT TO OTHERS

Though one may be overpowered, two can defend themselves. A cord of three strands is not quickly broken.

ECCLESIASTES 4:12

One of the commitments in First Place is to contact one person in your group each week. This may be in the form of a phone call, written note or an e-mail message. The most important reason for this commitment to encouragement is to reach out to others. When we begin First Place, we've already admitted that we have one problem in common—we need to learn to eat properly. We also need to learn to exercise and probably need a consistent Bible study and prayer time. Since we are aware of this common bond, reaching out to other group members becomes easier.

WHY SHOULD I ENCOURAGE OTHERS?

I have found that in church life, even in Sunday School, people have difficulty sharing their problems. We come to church on Sunday and when someone asks us how we are doing, we say "Fine." When we ask others how they are doing, they say "Fine," and we keep on going. If we ever need to say something besides "Fine," it's usually too late—our acquaintances have already gone down the hall, because they have places to go and things to do.

As members of a First Place group, we make time to be involved in each other's lives. We take the time to care. A contact during the week can make the difference in a person's day. It can say, "This group is different. In this group you can feel that someone cares enough to listen. You can share your joys and sorrows. We want to be here for you." It may be just the encouragement the person needs to stay on the program.

Some fear making the first contact. However, most have found this initial step opens a new door of opportunity and ministry. Keeping this commitment is so important. It's one tiny step toward reaching out to others who need your love.

People begin to see God's love when they see His love manifested in another human being. God's love becomes real to me when someone who shouldn't care about me, not only cares about me but also loves me. So don't neglect reaching out to others and encouraging them each week. Allow God to minister through and to you. It's as simple as picking up a phone or sending an e-mail. One of our leaders in Houston told about a time when this commitment meant very much to her.

My husband suffered a heart attack on a trip to visit our children in Waco. We were supposed to move my father into a nursing home in Dallas the same weekend. With my husband in ICU in a Waco hospital, our sons moved their grandfather into the nursing home and brought as many things as they could get into my car back to Waco. I then had to return to Houston with my father's things and make arrangements to store them and to get someone to take care of my classes at the Community College in order for me to be able to return to Waco to be with my husband. After a sleepless Sunday night and hectic Monday morning, I returned home to pack the car for the drive back to Waco. I listened to messages on the answering machine. The first call came from a member of my group. She knew nothing about what had transpired during the weekend. She said, "God laid you on my heart this morning. I felt that you needed special prayer and uplifting today. I just wanted you to know I'll be praying for you all day today. May God bless you." Those words of encouragement gave me the energy I needed to finish packing and make the three-hour drive back to Waco. I had been ready to cry and give up, but her phone call let me know I was never alone. Her prayers put "wind beneath my wings."

WHY IS REACHING OUT HARD FOR ME?

Reaching out and encouraging others through calling, writing or e-mailing is the one commitment that most First Place members find hard to do. Perhaps it is because we have been rejected and hurt many times in the past. We may have built walls around ourselves to keep people from ever hurting us again. I believe that God wants to begin emotional healing in each First Place member.

How to truly love other people is probably the most important thing that I have learned in the First Place program. I have learned how to love people that the world has said will never amount to anything—they'll never be useful, so why bother with them? I've grown up in a generation that says if people don't conform to what we tell them to do, then let's just forget about them. But God tells us something quite different. He says He loves every individual as much as He loves you and me. It doesn't matter what they've done. It doesn't matter what kind of sin they've committed.

God has taught me there are no degrees of sin. No sin is any worse than another, but all sin separates us from Him. And that's why it's so important that we not only confess our sin to Him but that we also reach out in love to those around us, that we forgive those who have sinned against us.

You're not going to be able to forgive overnight. But God, through your emotional healing, will empower you to forgive those who have sinned against you. When we refuse to forgive others, it's as if they were sitting in a chair strapped to our backs and we carry them all our lives. Our unforgiveness doesn't hurt them, but it hurts us tremendously.

I believe the root problem here is a lack of love. Perhaps we've never felt truly loved or never been able to totally love others. When the teachers of the Law asked Jesus what the greatest commandment is, He said to them, "'Love the Lord your God with all your heart and with all your soul and with all your mind and with all your strength.' The second is this: 'Love your neighbor as yourself.' There is no commandment greater than these'" (Mark 12:30,31). This command is repeated in three of the Gospels. We need to realize that if Jesus said it was the greatest commandment, then He meant it.

I think many of us have a problem accepting and showing love. We may not have received enough love as children, or we didn't receive unconditional love from our parents, teachers or other significant people in our lives. As a result, loving ourselves, as well as God, may be difficult. We may find God's unconditional love, as described throughout Scripture, difficult to comprehend. Therefore, reaching out and loving others is difficult for us. When we are filled with God's love, we are able to love others (see 1 John 4:21).

As we continue in the First Place program, we will learn how God truly loves us just the way we are. However, God is committed to conforming us to the image of His Son, Jesus. In doing so, some changes will occur. We have to make the choice to change. We have to choose the things that are talked about in this book. And we have to choose them on a daily basis, so God can make the changes.

If reaching out to other people because you've been hurt in the past is difficult, then you need to pray for God to show you one person in your group whom you can trust. Ask God to help you bond with one person to whom you can reach out and who will love you back. God will honor your request. He'll begin to teach you about His love. As He demonstrates His love through others around you, He's going to give you the courage to trust and love in return.

WHAT DO I SAY?

When you reach out to another First Place member, you already know you have a common interest. You can always begin with a typical First Place question, "How is your week going?" The one you contact may be having a good week, and the two of you can celebrate. If not, don't feel that you have to fix problems or make the week a success. Just listening and caring will mean a lot. If you have a suggestion to share, do so in a way that leaves the other person free to accept it or not.

Reaching out enables you to be aware of what's going on in the other person's life. This sharing will not always happen the first time but comes as you cultivate trust and friendship. Often, we may feel the food temptations we have are greater than those of anyone else; or we may feel no one would understand the experiences we've had in life, because no one has been through anything like we have. Personal contact helps us realize that other people have suffered just like we have suffered and that they are struggling in the same areas. We discover how God has healed others and is continuing to heal. As we are healed, we can be a part of the process of healing for others.

We have people tell us they had a cookie or a piece of cake in their hand just when someone from their group called. Some have put the caller on hold while they disposed of a cookie. That's the way the Holy Spirit works. The Holy Spirit will urge us to reach out to someone. Many times you will contact someone and he or she will say, "I am so glad you called. You don't know what I'm going through right now." Or someone will call you when you are having a particularly difficult day.

Pray for the person before you contact him or her, but don't neglect to pray together and praise God for working through both of you. Frequent prayer is a habit I learned from a friend in Atlanta a few years ago. I never talk to her on the phone that she doesn't say, "Well, let's pray together before we hang up." It has been such a blessing to me to pray with fellow Christians.

I hope you will pray with the person you contact. If you're on the phone, you can say, "Could we just pray together before we hang up?" If you're writing a note or e-mail message, you can include a short prayer and Scripture. Ask God to bless that person and wrap His arms around him or her that day. Allow the other person to pray for you, too. I never fail to be uplifted when I hear someone interceding for me, taking my name and my needs to God in prayer.

Prayer is such an important part of my life today, and I never start a meeting without praying first. Nor do I go into a counseling situation without having everyone involved pray together at the beginning and the end of the session. God blesses our lives when we ask Him. He wants His children to come to Him and petition Him, so don't neglect praying together with the people in your group. Praise God after the meeting is over for the things He has accomplished during your time together.

HOW DOES REACHING OUT TO OTHERS HELP ME?

I believe God wants to use men and women who have suffered terribly and have begun to heal to minister to others. I believe God was there when they were enduring such pain. He loves them so much that He will not only heal them but also use them in the very same area where they have suffered.

I see men and women today who have been healed or who are being healed of some form of abuse, reaching out to other men and women who have been abused and loving them through Christ. I see people who are struggling with a health condition being strengthened by others with the same condition.

You might not realize it now, but encouraging others is a wonderful way to receive encouragement. You can take heart in knowing that someone else experiences your temptations, your failures. You can have hope for yourself when you see that someone else has overcome those temptations, has turned failures into success. Encouragement is a twofold blessing: it blesses the one giving and the one receiving.

So don't be afraid to reach out to others. See in them the struggles that you share. See in them the joy and the peace that living out First Place can bring. Encourage them—and you will be encouraged!

CHOOSING TO PRAY

Pray without ceasing.

1 THESSALONIANS 5:17, KJV

Prayer is the third commitment of the First Place program. Everything that we do should be bathed in prayer. God wants His children to pray. With my own children, there are many things I would have done for them or given to them if only they had asked. I have to believe that our heavenly Father feels the same way about us. He wants us to come to Him and express our needs, our worries and our problems and allow Him to help us. Prayer is such an important part of balance in our lives. In First Place, we want you to set aside quiet time each day so that you can be alone with the Lord in prayer.

DEVELOPING THE HABIT

Before I began First Place, I didn't have a regular quiet time. I used to rely on "shoot-up praying." When someone came into my office for counsel, I would silently pray, "Lord, you know her needs; lead me to help her just now." I have found that the more time I spend in prayer during my quiet time, the less often I need to rely solely on spontaneous shoot-up praying. I am more aware of what is happening around me, and I look for God to speak to others through me.

When I spend time with God daily, He conditions my heart ahead of time to meet the needs of people I come in contact with each day. Psalm 32:8 says, "I will instruct you and teach you in the way you should go; I will counsel you and watch over you." What a promise! Of course, we don't want to go through life without instruction, nor do we want to reject the promise of a counselor and someone to watch over us.

Jesus is our example of a prayerful life. He spent much time praying alone and in a quiet place. One biblical example is found in Luke 5:16, "Jesus often withdrew to lonely places and prayed." Obviously, He knew the value of not being distracted. We see the evidence of prayer in His life through His close relationship with the Father, His sinless life, His power in accomplishing the Father's will and His commitment to follow God no matter the cost.

Prayer gives us access to the Creator of the universe, who loves us so much that He instituted prayer as a way to personally communicate with each of His children. Prayer is God's idea. I pray because I need and want to, but I also pray because God desires communion with me.

USING A PRAYER JOURNAL

Writing my prayers helps me stay focused during my prayer time. Previously, I could not pray for even five minutes without thoughts of the day ahead distracting me. Many times I was thinking about what I was going to eat for breakfast, what I would do when I got to work and what was planned for that evening. Perhaps you have had this experience of setting aside a quiet time and being disappointed when you realize you have spent that time with your mind on everything except the Lord.

Over and over, I kept trying to establish a daily quiet time. I attended every prayer seminar that came along. Finally, I discovered my answer. I keep my focus on the Lord during my quiet time by writing my prayers in a journal. This approach works for me and I recommend it to you.

When I started my first prayer journal in 1990, I thought I didn't need to include Sunday in my journal because I went to church. I have since learned that Sunday is a very important day for me to get up early to spend time with my heavenly Father. Sunday morning quiet time prepares me by establishing an attitude of worship and expectancy so that I am ready for all that God will do on His day. Now I try to journal every day. Your prayer journal will become a daily habit as you commit to making it an important part of your prayer time.

Another advantage of keeping a prayer journal is being able to see how God answers prayer—even when you don't realize why you're praying for a certain person or thing. One morning during my quiet time, I felt led to pray for one of our leaders from another church. When I got to work that morning, I sent her a note and told her that I didn't know why she was on my heart that morning, but I had prayed for her. About a week later, I received a letter saying, "You will never know what it meant to know that you were praying for me that day. It was a witness to my spirit that the Holy Spirit impressed you to pray." She shared with me all the events that were going on in her life that day and how much turmoil she was in. The Holy Spirit has the power to unite believers through the power of prayer. We need to show up for our prayer time each day to allow God to communicate to us the people that need our prayers.

Irene Bonner of Georgia says the discipline of writing her prayers in a prayer journal has been one of the most meaningful parts of the program for her. "I go back with a red pen and highlight in my journal ways God has answered my prayers. I have learned to commit minor things to Him as well as major things. I have learned that if something bothers me, it bothers Him, too."

Praying for Yourself

We should never feel guilty about praying for our own needs. The model prayer (see Matt. 6:9-13) teaches us to ask for our daily bread. Some of our needs are minor or routine; others may be dramatic.

In the early days of the program, Dottie Brewer, the first director of First Place, was involved in a serious hit-and-run automobile accident. Her car caught on fire. She tried to open the door on the driver's side but could not. She yelled out, "Help me!" to God. Immediately the passenger-side door flew open and a man dressed completely in white pulled her out of the car just before it exploded. The man never said a word. Dottie watched the car explode. When she turned around, the man was gone. Dottie had no doubt that God had sent an angel to rescue her from that burning car. Dottie said, "I sure was glad God and I had such a close relationship that I only had to cry out, 'help me.' God knew immediately it was me and sent help."

Dottie was in the hospital for several days following the accident. Before the accident, Dottie had finished the manuscript for the original leader's guide for First Place but had not sent it to the publisher. The people in the First Place office didn't have the heart to tell her the only copy of that leader's guide had been in her car when it burned.

When she was well enough, Dottie's husband, Foster, took her to see the car, which had been totaled. The leader's guide manuscript was in the trunk. Everything in the guide had burned except the logo on the front cover. As Dottie examined the manuscript, she saw that there was enough writing on each page (just the size of that logo) to make her believe that she could reconstruct the guide.

During the Thanksgiving holiday following the accident, while her husband and son went deer hunting, Dottie spread those charred pages out on her living-room floor and began to reconstruct the leader's guide—all from about 15 words in the center of each page! There is no doubt in our minds that just as God had preserved her life, He also preserved the work that she had done. One verse that we memorize in First Place is Jeremiah 29:11, "'For I know the plans I have for you,' declares the LORD, 'plans to prosper you and not to harm you, plans to give you hope and a future.'"

PRAYING FOR OTHERS

When Sharon Norris of Houston was laid off from her job, she asked her First Place group to pray for her. "That next Tuesday night in class my instructor prayed with me to give me peace and comfort of mind that I would be OK. I was so happy that someone cared so much to pray for me that day." Prayer for others unites us to them in the power of the Holy Spirit.

Praying for others also invites the Lord into our relationships with them. Sometimes we need to talk to God about relationships. Strained relationships appear in families, neighborhoods, work situations, church or anywhere else we interact with other people. We can accomplish far more by talking to God than going to that person and "trying to straighten him or her out." We may think we know the answer to a problem, but the other person may not accept that answer from us. God must be our guide in the matter of timing. We can avoid having to confront other people, if we spend time in prayer and wait for God to do His work.

One of our leaders related the following incident:

Our son and family moved to a different town. Several weeks went by, but they made no effort to find a new church home. We prayed daily about this. We were wondering how long we should wait before saying anything and how we could say something tactfully. We decided to wait until the Lord led us to mention our concern. Then these welcome words came from our son, "The little church down the road has church at 11 o'clock and we'll be there next Sunday. We were going to attend last Sunday, but when we got in the car, the battery was dead."

The Lord answers your prayers for others in His time. You must be patient and faithful in waiting on the Lord. God has a plan for all of us, so entrust your concerns for others to Him in prayer.

At First Place we have experienced firsthand—and in a quite humorous way—how God answers our prayers by revealing His plans. One of our leaders felt led to quit work, so she could stay home with her teenagers, and she asked us to pray for her situation. Several months later she received a rather unexpected answer to her prayer. She became pregnant with her fourth child! We jokingly told her that she needed to be more specific with us when she asked us to pray.

USING SCRIPTURE IN PRAYER

We can find so many ways to pray for others, but what better method than to include His Word in your prayers? Scripture plays an important role in my prayers for my loved ones. When I pray for others, I often use Philippians 1:3-6:

> I thank my God every time I remember you. In all my prayers for all of you, I always pray with joy because of your partnership in the gospel from the first day until now, being confident of this, that he who began a good work in you will carry it on to completion until the day of Christ Jesus.

I have found quoting Scripture is an effective way to pray. And I am confident that you will, too. If you have never prayed using Scripture, now is a great time to start. In fact, the last two days of each week of your Bible studies address this technique and give good examples of Scripture-based prayers.

PRAYING ALOUD

You may be concerned about being asked to pray aloud in your group. If so, share your concern with your leader. You may want to ask your leader or a trusted friend in the group to allow you to practice praying with him or her until you feel confident to pray in the group. No one is asked to pray aloud unless he or she is comfortable doing so. If you are comfortable praying aloud, you may feel led to help another group member who may be struggling with this point.

GIVING PRAYER PRIORITY

Daily prayer is essential. To come before our heavenly Father each day, whether we feel like it or not, is an act of obedience. We tend to treat our friends so much better than we treat our heavenly Father. We check on our friends, spend time with them, listen to them and ask their advice. How often do we listen to the advice of God?

Phyllis Lincer of Canada wrote us, "I had let my time alone with God deteriorate in recent years. I was no longer diligent about setting aside time to meet with my Lord each morning. My focus was no longer on Christ. As I began to really listen with my heart, I realized that my heart had shifted away from Him." Fortunately, by establishing a regular quiet time, Phyllis reported that God's grace overwhelmed her and she was able to give control to the Father.

Kathy Smith of Nebraska reminds us, "I'm driven to pray because I know that I'm very vulnerable; and without daily communication with my God—basically His convicting and my giving in to Him—I will fail."

We can only first seek God's kingdom by keeping in touch with the King! I hope that a meaningful daily experience with prayer will be one of the greatest blessings that will grow out of your First Place participation.

CHOOSING TO READ GOD'S WORD

All Scripture is God-breathed and is useful for teaching, rebuking, correcting and training in righteousness, so that the man of God may be thoroughly equipped for every good work.

2 TIMOTHY 3:16,17

Scripture reading is the fourth commitment in the First Place program. We ask you to read at least two chapters of God's Word each day. You will have lists of Scriptures from the Old and New Testaments to work from. Our purpose is to encourage you to read God's Word daily.

A LOVE LETTER

When I was 16, my parents took me on a summer vacation to Yellowstone National Park. I was in love and didn't want to be away from my boyfriend, Johnny, whom I would later marry. He had promised to send letters to me along the way. My parents took me to all the general delivery post offices in Yellowstone to let me check for letters from Johnny. When a letter came, I was so excited to hear how much he was missing me and to keep up with all that was going on at home. A couple of years ago, I found those letters while looking through some old high school memorabilia. It was touching to read again the words, written so many years ago, of the one who loves me so very much, even to this day.

If people can love us so much, how much more does God, whose love is infinite and perfect? God's Word is a love letter that was written long ago to you and me. Read John 3:16 with your name inserted in place of the words "the world." You will be reminded of how much God loves you.

A Guide for Daily Living

The Bible, God's letter to me, gives me instruction. It leads me in the right direction. It teaches me right from wrong. God's Word contains instruction on how to raise and discipline my children. It contains instruction on how to overcome bad habits by being more disciplined. Everything that an individual would ever need in life is found in God's Word—a reality we affirm in all aspects of the First Place program.

As you read God's Word, apply it to your daily life. Applying it may mean that you will stop reading when a particular verse speaks to you. Many can bear witness, as perhaps you can, that while reading a familiar passage, suddenly it becomes real to you and applies to what is happening in your life. One leader wrote,

> Recently I experienced a back problem. While reading Psalm 38:7 my heart pounded faster. The verse read, "My back is filled with searing pain." This verse had not meant much to me previously. At other times I would have continued reading without a pause. But this time as I continued to read, I felt the writing was very personal.

As we strive to overcome deeply instilled habits and addictions, this love letter gives us confidence, hope and vision. A verse that has meant much to me is 1 John 4:4, "You, dear children, are from God and have overcome them, because the one who is in you is greater than the one who is in the world." When you feel your heart quickened by the Holy Spirit, search His Word to find something that will help you today to serve Him better. As a Scripture verse becomes a part of you, you will be able to use it to help others.

A Meditation

Meditating on what we read is important. Internalizing Scripture reveals what it means for us, personally. When I was running, I loved to meditate on God's Word by using Scripture music audiocassettes as I ran each morning. The music was such a blessing to my life each day. I enjoyed these cassettes so much that I believe God used the experience to place the dream in my heart of having our own First Place Scripture memory audiocassettes/CDs as a part of the program. Today this dream has become a reality and although I can no longer run for exercise, I now listen to our First Place Scripture CDs as I walk, ride a bicycle or drive my car to and from work.

Audiocassettes of the Bible are another way of meditating on Scripture. While in your car, you can listen to God's Word being read. Jesus promised in John 14:26 that the Holy Spirit would remind us of the things He has taught us. I am often amazed at how true this is: Many nights, I awake in the middle of the night and realize I am singing Scripture memory verses as I lie half asleep. As we take in God's Word, it stays in our subconscious. It becomes part of us. Then the Holy Spirit recalls Scripture for us when we need it. That's why it's so essential for us to fill ourselves with God's Word.

Reading Scripture and listening to it are also important when we realize the influence of the information we take in and process daily. Much of what we see and hear in the world will lead us to doubt, worry and disillusionment. Yet page after page of the Bible gives us hope, peace and comfort. Always remember the gentle words of Jesus in John 14:27:

> Peace I leave with you; my peace I give you. I do not give to you as the world gives. Do not let your hearts be troubled and do not be afraid.

So fear no more. The Lord is walking with you as you choose to read His Word and give Him first place in your life. He who has overcome the world will enable you to overcome every obstacle that is keeping you from living the balanced life He wants for you.

CHOOSING TO MEMORIZE GOD'S WORD

I have hidden your word in my heart that I might not sin against you.

PSALM 119:11

In First Place we strive to bring discipline into an undisciplined life. One way to cultivate discipline is to memorize one verse of the Bible study each week. That is only 10 verses to memorize in 10 weeks. We quote each verse from memory as we weigh in at the beginning of each session.

GOD USES SCRIPTURE MEMORY TO ENCOURAGE US

Memorizing God's Word assures us that when we have a need, the Holy Spirit will comfort us with His Word. His promise is found in John 14:26: "The Counselor, the Holy Spirit, whom the Father will send in my name, will teach you all things and will remind you of everything I have said to you." Many times I have parts of verses in my head but don't know the references, so I have to look them up in a concordance. During times of extreme need, I may not have time to do that.

I heard a story about a lady who kept asking God to give her a verse to help her cope with her stressful week. When she didn't receive a verse, she sought the aid of her pastor. After she quoted the Scriptures she knew, he observed, "Well, of the three verses you have memorized, none of them applies." This lady didn't have enough verses committed to memory to know God's mind regarding her particular need. So the first reason for memorizing God's Word is that it provides resources from which the Holy Spirit may draw in our time of need.

Scripture memorization also enables us to resist temptation. When I go to the grocery store, I am lured over to the bakery area. I know that I'm not going to purchase anything there; I just want to look at it and lust after it. I cannot tell you how many times I have stood there looking in the bakery cases when this particular First Place Scripture memory verse comes to my mind: "No temptation has seized you except what is common to man. And God is faithful; he will not let you be tempted beyond what you can bear" (1 Cor. 10:13). I memorized that verse when I joined First Place. It has served me well by reminding me that even when I am tempted, God is faithful. All I have to do is ask, and He will give me the strength to resist that temptation.

You will find that many of the verses we memorize in First Place are able to guide us in controlling our eating. Jesus' example during His 40 days of temptation reminds us that "Man does not live on bread alone" (Matt. 4:4). This verse helps when we may be tempted to use food to meet a need, when physical hunger is not the need.

Lastly, His Word reminds us that He is beside us each day—we cannot hide from Him. As many people do, I have tried to tell myself that if no one sees me eat it, it won't count. But I know that though no one else may know what I eat, God does and so do I. The words of Psalm 69:5 remind us, "You know my folly, O God; my guilt is not hidden from you." Remember, too, that He is there, not as a policeman but as your loving Father. Being reminded that He is present should be a tremendous consolation to us: we are never alone.

GOD USES SCRIPTURE MEMORY TO ENCOURAGE OTHERS

Memorizing God's Word is one of the most important commitments of the First Place program—a fact we emphasize throughout the program. In fact, at the beginning of youth camp one year, our youth minister confiscated every piece of Scripture that the kids had. He locked away all the Bibles. The only Scripture the youths had was what they had committed to memory. During that week, they tried to reconstruct their Bible from memory. This was a very sobering experience for them. They realized the necessity of Scripture memorization.

Paul tells us in Romans 10:17, "Faith comes from hearing the message, and the message is heard through the word of Christ." I believe memorizing Scripture is a commitment we usually don't take seriously enough. We may not realize what God can do with His Word. The Holy Spirit can bring it to mind when we are ministering to others. When we're talking to others who have a need, our helping them takes on a spiritual dimension when we can say "You know, it says in God's Word . . ." and quote a relevant Scripture for them. Our help to others is based on how God works through us. Without His words and power, we may leave a friend no better off than before we shared our counsel.

Memorization can involve family members who are not involved with Bible study or Scripture memory. Ask a family member to check while you recite your memory verse. You may want to stumble a bit and ask that person to read it to you. One of our First Place leaders has a husband who doesn't know Christ, but he is willing to listen to her recite her memory verse to help her. He doesn't realize how God can use his hearing these verses to lead him to faith in Christ.

Children and teenagers are often challenged to do what mom or dad is doing. Try memorizing a chapter, and you may need lots of help from the family! Your helper may be memorizing without knowing it. A few years ago, my associate Kay Smith wanted to learn Psalm 19. She practiced the psalm everywhere she went. She said it to her grandsons while driving in the car. She said it to me when we were on First Place trips together. The worst part was, each time she made a mistake, she would start over at the beginning! We all got to where we prayed for a perfect recitation the first time around! We laughed about her reciting the chapter so much, but I never hear or read Psalm 19 that I don't think of Kay.

God will put the desire in your heart to memorize more and more of His Word. The most effective people I know in the Christian world have a vast knowledge of Scripture that allows God to work through them.

GOD ENABLES US TO MEMORIZE SCRIPTURE

I have heard individuals say that they just can't memorize. Martha Norsworthy of Kentucky wrote us to say, "Since adulthood, I had not been successful in memorizing Scripture, but the First Place Scriptures ministered to me in such a way that I was able to memorize them. Through First Place, God began to do a great work in my life."

Personally I find it helpful to use the First Place Scripture memory audiocassettes and CDs. Hearing Scripture put to music plants it in my mind as I listen. Children are often taught the ABCs by singing them. Numbers are taught by singing a song about them. You remember commercials that have a catchy tune. In fact, I can recall some I have not heard for at least 20 years; I would have forgotten the words, but I can still recite them because of the tune that accompanied them. If you will plant Scriptures in your mind, God will remind you of them.

Take in Scripture as often as you can. We most certainly should use our minds to absorb God's Word to us. Remember Peter's admonition: "Prepare your minds for action; be self-controlled; set your hope fully on the grace to be given you when Jesus Christ is revealed" (1 Pet. 1:13).

In the mornings after I have exercised at our Christian Life Center, I like to recall the memory verse for the week as I am getting dressed. Then I try to recall all of the verses I have learned so far in the study. This practice keeps them in my mind and heart as I memorize the current week's verse. We're told we have to do something for 21 days for it to become a habit. This also applies to Scripture memorization. We have to make it ours. We have to make it personal.

I meet so many people, but I have a difficult time remembering names. If I memorize something about them, something about their facial characteristics to go along with their names, it helps me to bring up a mental picture of them. In turn, I am able to remember their names. In the same way, I try to lock in something from the verse I am memorizing—a mental picture, a colorful verb—that helps me recall it.

God will not make us memorize Scripture. We have to be obedient. We begin by memorizing one verse a week.

If you feel that this commitment is too difficult, that you couldn't possibly memorize a verse each week, ask the Lord to help you. He will enable you to commit His Word to memory. With His help, you will not consider Scripture memorization a chore. Rather, you will see it for what it truly is—a great gift to yourself.

Marge Watson of Kentucky sums up the blessings Bible study and Scripture memorization have been to her when she says, "Although the journey for weight loss may come to an end, I hope I never reach the end of my spiritual journey. My Bible studies and verses in First Place have been a blessing."

Memorization is a very valuable tool in the Christian life, and God will use it in a mighty way if we will choose to memorize His Word.

CHOOSING TO STUDY GOD'S WORD

Do your best to present yourself to God as one approved, a workman who does not need to be ashamed and who correctly handles the word of truth.

2 TIMOTHY 2:15

The First Place Bible studies consist of 10 weeks of study, with each study divided into seven days—one for each day of the week. The first five days involve Scriptures, questions and interactive learning activities and take no longer than 10 to 15 minutes to complete. After you read a Scripture passage, you will apply it to your life by responding through use of activities such as matching exercises, filling in the blanks or writing a Scripture verse in your own words. Days 6 and 7 are a time to reflect on what you have learned for the week. These two days conclude with examples of Scriptures put into prayer form, but they also give you time to think about your memory verse and provide tips on memorizing Scripture and praying. This method of teaching has been used in Bible study materials for many years. When you have completed a Bible study, it is your book, a record of what happened in your life as you studied God's Word for a 10-week period.

When you come to the weekly group meeting and go over the Bible study with your leader and other group members, you will find that God has spoken to each person according to his or her need. He will say amazingly different things to each one of you through His Word. Your life will be enriched as you hear from group members, and you will enrich their lives as you share with them your experiences with God's Word during the week.

RESOURCES FOR STUDYING GOD'S WORD

As I grow in my Christian life, I hunger to study God's Word. If you are just becoming a student of God's Word, I have several suggestions for you. Begin to acquire the following books to enhance your Bible study. You may need to do so over a period of time. And remember that these books make good presents to give and receive.

- *The translation of the Bible most familiar to you.* There are many translations of the Bible. Although First Place Bible studies, Scripture memory verses and Scripture memory songs are based on the *New International Version*, you may enjoy the *King James Version* while someone else might enjoy the *American Standard Bible* or the *New Living Translation*.

- *A parallel Bible (a Bible with four or more translations).* This tool is useful for comparing the different translations and getting a feel for what each verse means.

- *An unabridged concordance.* An alphabetized list of words from the Bible, a concordance will help you find a verse or subject that you want to study. For example, if you are experiencing fear or worry in your life and want to know what the Bible has to say about it, look up the word "fear" in the concordance. A concordance will show you every time that word is mentioned in the Bible. As you study the Scriptures using the information you find in the concordance, you will survey the wealth of knowledge that God has revealed to us.

- *A Bible commentary.* Commentaries are like encyclopedias on the Bible. They may be found in one volume, two volumes or multiple-volume sets. A commentary explains to you what a verse or passage means in the context of what was going on at the time it was written. It explains keywords in their original language. The commentary writer, a Bible scholar, gives his opinion—as well as the opinions of other Bible scholars—regarding the meaning of a verse or chapter. As a result of reading a commentary, you have a broader understanding of the passage you are studying.

• *An encyclopedia*. While preparing to teach a Sunday School lesson on fear, I came across 1 Peter 5:8: "Be self-controlled and alert. Your enemy the devil prowls around like a roaring lion looking for someone to devour." God used that verse to help me understand that fear is as real as if a person were standing in the presence of a lion. I consulted an encyclopedia for the characteristics of lions: Lions attack at night. They attack animals that are weaker. The oldest lion with the loudest roar prowls one side of a clearing, while the youngest, fiercest lions roam the other side of the clearing. The older lion then begins to roar. When the animals run away from the roar, they run right into the jaws of the young lions. This deception seals the fate of the fleeing animals. Fear has led to their deaths. Fear is not from God; it is from our enemy.

• *A Bible dictionary*. With a Bible dictionary you will be able to define terms such as "sanctification" and "atonement."

You might not think you have the resources to invest in all of these Bible study materials. Most study Bibles have an abridged concordance and Bible maps. Others include a glossary, or dictionary. A good study Bible will get you started on your journey of in-depth Bible study.

There are also Bible software programs available which include all of the tools listed above. Such a program is well worth the investment if you desire to become a student of the Bible.

If after completing your daily Bible study in First Place, you find yourself wanting more, do an in-depth study of the key verse for that day or of a passage used in that day's study. Find the meaning of the original Greek or Hebrew words or follow the cross-references provided.

If you do just a small amount of research each day, by the end of the week you will have had an enriching study of God's Word.

An Appetite for Bible Study

Can you remember a food that you disliked as a child? Did you find when you became an adult that the food tasted different? Now you like it. Some people don't like Bible study for a number of reasons. They may have disliked school, and Bible study reminds them of their homework assignments. Perhaps they thought of the Bible as too difficult, because they had never read the newer translations. Maybe the Bible had been used as a scare tactic to keep them from disobeying. If you are one of those who speaks of Bible study and spinach or broccoli in the same breath, you may have to develop a taste for Bible study.

Bible study does not come naturally. The devil doesn't want us reading the truth. He will do everything possible to keep us from the Bible. When I joined First Place, I was not involved in regular personal Bible study. The First Place Bible study was the starting point for me.

Studying God's Word will become easier for you as you set aside a regular study time. Hours formerly spent watching television or reading the newspaper or magazines may become devoted to reading, studying and memorizing God's Word. Studying God's Word will be the most beneficial use you'll ever make of your time.

As you study the Bible, His Word will be clearer to you. You will learn to look forward to your study time. Like any appetite, it must be fed in order to grow. Feed your Bible study appetite, and watch the Lord use this time to bless your life.

Benefits of Bible Study to First Place

God has told us of the power of His Word. The writer of Hebrews expressed that power this way, "The word of God is living and active. Sharper than any double-edged sword, it penetrates even to dividing soul and spirit, joints and marrow; it judges the thoughts and attitudes of the heart" (Heb. 4:12). This is the power that enables us to change our attitude about God, our lives and other human beings as well as our attitudes about food. No wonder lives are changed through daily Bible study.

Keeping the commitment to study the Bible will not only help you develop spiritual muscles but will also change your attitude toward food and exercise, starting you down the road to a new lifestyle. Many people come into First Place blaming someone else for their extra weight. As this "living and active" word "judges the thoughts and attitudes," individuals begin to take responsibility for their own choices. They are empowered to make a change. Improved relationships with family members and friends are often the result. Temper control, total honesty, patience and compassion are other positive outcomes.

As Jim Clayton of Tennessee expresses it, "First Place has completely changed my life, and God continues to do some remarkable things as I yield myself more and more to Him. Each day is more exciting, as I share what He is doing."

CHOOSING TO EAT RIGHT

Do you not know that your body is a temple of the Holy Spirit, who is in you,
whom you have received from God? You are not your own; you were bought at a
price. Therefore honor God with your body.

1 CORINTHIANS 6:19,20

Food is an everyday concern. We have three meals a day. (Some of us eat many more times than that!) We can't quit eating.

Making good food choices doesn't make you a good person, and neither does making a bad choice make you a bad person. Most of you have come into First Place with enough guilt to last a lifetime. We don't want to heap more guilt on you for what you eat or do not eat.

Our purpose is to help you realize that God is the one who will change your life as you trust Him every day and as you ask Him to make those changes. We have to choose to live a lifestyle that will be pleasing to God. Serving God as long as we can, as well as we can, is the best motivation for wanting to practice good nutrition. Other motivations, such as health concerns, may or may not last a lifetime.

MOTIVATIONS FOR EATING RIGHT

We each have different reasons for wanting to keep the seventh commitment of First Place. These reasons fall into three general categories:

- We want to lose weight.
- We have health concerns.
- We want to practice good nutrition.

Let's examine each of these areas of interest.

We Want to Lose Weight

For some of us the need is to lose weight. When I started First Place, the only reason I wanted to lose weight was to improve my physical appearance. I was approaching my 40th birthday, and I didn't want to look 40 when I got there. Even though my motivation was not biblical, God was working in my life. He wanted my body to glorify Him as a discipled believer.

You may have joined First Place through the coaxing of your spouse. If your motivation is not coming from within yourself, you may find difficulty in staying with the program. If you have not joined a First Place group on your own initiative, pray that God will allow you to see the benefits of First Place and therefore change your outlook to a more positive one. If your goal is to be a certain size for a class reunion, wedding or special event, after the occasion takes place, you may have no motivation to persist in the program. In this case, you will most likely go back to your former habits. If you do, the weight will return.

We who have weight problems eat for many reasons. We eat when we're happy, when we're sad, when we're depressed or when we're anxious. We have so many excuses to eat. God not only wants to change what we eat, but He also wants to change why we eat. If you have a tremendous amount of weight to lose, find out why you are eating more than you should.

Losing weight will be the result of changes in eating habits and lifestyle. The rewards are great when you get to your goal. First Place has many leaders across the United States who have lost over 100 pounds, and the difference that it has made in their lives is gratifying. One leader told me that walking down the aisle of a bus without having to turn sideways, and sitting in a movie theater without getting bruises from the sides of the chair, mean so much to her. Many of us who don't have that kind of weight to lose don't understand what those victories mean in a life.

When you begin First Place, you will be asked to set a weight-loss goal for the 13-week session. Using the Live-It food plan, women will be consuming no less than 1,400 calories a day and men, 1,800. On this plan you will probably lose a pound and a half to two pounds a week. We know that it's not possible to lose any more fat than that each week. If you were to lose more weight than that every week by eating fewer calories, you would lose lean body mass along with the fat. We definitely do not want you to lose lean body mass. Lean body mass is your bones, organs and muscles. It gives you the energy to do the things that you need to do every day. In First Place most people lose 20 to 25 pounds in 13 weeks.

You can repeat this 13-week cycle until you reach your lifetime goal. If you have over 50 pounds to lose, we encourage you to initially increase the number of calories used in our Live-It food plan. Women can eat from 1,500 to 1,800 calories a day and men from 2,000 to 2,600 calories a day. If you have quite a bit of weight to lose, usually you'll lose at the same rate of one and a half to two pounds a week, even on more calories. The indicator is whether you are truly hungry. We want you to have enough calories so that you will not be hungry, because hunger is what causes you to want to go off any program after a short period of time.

An inadequate variety of foods will also prompt you to leave a diet program. Many diets allow little variety as far as the types of food you can eat. In First Place you will be able to choose from a great variety of wonderful foods, so you will not get bored with the program and want to quit. You cannot fail First Place. You can quit. You can stop doing it. But you cannot fail, because the success is in the process of First Place.

God wants every one of us to be able to serve Him as long as we can, as best we can. Begin to pray that God will change your appetite so that you will desire food that is good for your body. Ask God to direct your motive for wanting to lose weight so that you can have a lifestyle change. Unless you have a lifestyle change, you are destined to gain this weight over and over again.

We Have Health Concerns

Some of us have health concerns that require a specialized diet. Though not always the cause, poor health sometimes results from poor nutrition. The psalmist said, "You created my inmost being. . . . I praise you because I am fearfully and wonderfully made" (Ps. 139:13,14). As you reflect upon the magnificent body God has given you, you begin to realize that the food you put into your body is very important.

Proper nutrition is the key to keeping your body strong and healthy. In First Place, there are no gimmicks, just a healthy way to eat. We use the USDA Food Pyramid in the First Place program. Our food plan uses an exchange system endorsed by the American Dietetic Association and the American Heart Association.

We want to learn to eat properly because, as Americans, we lead the world in these five major health problems:

- Cancer
- Heart disease
- Diabetes
- Hypertension, or high blood pressure
- Lower back pain

Dr. Dick Couey, author and professor of nutrition and fitness, tells us that the reason we suffer from these five major health problems is because of our eating habits and our sedentary lifestyle. We lead the world in colon cancer because Americans eat such a small amount of fiber. Most of us eat about four grams of fiber a day, as opposed to the recommended 25 to 35 grams. In First Place you will learn what foods are high in fiber, so you can incorporate them into your daily food plan.

Diabetes is called the Silent Killer. Many diabetics don't know they are diabetic until they go to the doctor for another problem. An Ohio pastor who is diabetic relates in his testimony how he discovered First Place when his wife started a First Place group. When he heard about the food plan, he said, "Well, I know all about that. I'm a diabetic and I've seen the dietitian teach proper eating using these food modules that you use." He not only lost 36 pounds but also was able to stop taking all but one of his diabetes medications.

He and many other Americans are Type 2 diabetics—people who develop the disease later in life. Type 2 diabetics respond very quickly to proper nutrition and exercise. If you are a diabetic, we encourage you to adopt this lifestyle change for the rest of your life. As you begin to practice good health through the support of First Place, we hope you will experience a radical change in the area of good health and that you will be able to eventually eliminate many of the medications you are taking today.

We have heard that sugar does not cause diabetes if eaten in the right amounts. But sugar is hidden in many prepared foods. In the early 1900s, Americans ate 6 pounds of sugar a year. Americans in the twenty-first century eat 140 pounds of sugar a year.[1] You may think *Well, I don't eat that much sugar.* Are you sure? A cola drink contains 10 to 12 teaspoons of sugar and a piece of chocolate cake contains 12 to 14 teaspoons.

Maybe you have switched to low-fat desserts, because you know you need to cut your fat intake and lower your cholesterol. Many food companies have come to the rescue by cutting the amount of fat in their products. Many foods now come in two forms: regular and lite, or low fat. Consumers buy and eat these low-fat products that taste as good or almost as good as the regular recipe. But to be palatable to the consumer, more sugar has been added. As our sugar intake reaches a new high, leaders in the health field fear that Type 2 diabetes among Americans will increase and start showing itself at an earlier age.

When we enter First Place, we are asked to watch our sugar intake until we get to our goal weight. We believe in following the recommendations of the major health organizations. Sugar is neither a "good" food nor a "bad" food. However, when it comes to a healthy eating plan, sugar provides calories but little nutrition. When trying to achieve and maintain a healthy weight, it's a good idea to cut back on sugar in favor of more nutritious foods, such as fruits, vegetables and whole grains. Many First Place members have found success by strictly limiting processed sugar in their eating plan. If a member is meeting his or her body's nutritional needs and maintaining a healthy weight, moderate amounts of sugar can be included in the eating plan. You have to decide what's best for you. While not addictive, sugar does trigger binge eating in some individuals.

We also encourage you to remember moderation when using artificial sweeteners. You can get a tremendous amount of artificial sugar in a day's time if you drink a lot of diet drinks and eat sugar-free pudding or yogurt. We don't want you to put too much of anything artificial into your body. Whether you have an illness as a result of poor eating, lack of exercise or hereditary factors, good nutrition will improve your overall health and enable your body to serve you as best it can.

We Want to Practice Good Nutrition

Our busy lifestyles have led us to rely on fast foods and frozen dinners. Fat content is high in many of these and, unfortunately, even the health-iest frozen dinners are high in sodium. If you plan ahead, home-cooked meals can be prepared just as quickly and at a much lower cost. The main rule to remember in the First Place Live-It plan is to avoid process-ed foods as much as possible and eat fresh foods—fruits, vegetables, meats, whole-grain breads. The American Heart Association recom-mends eating cold-water fatty fish at least twice a week to obtain omega-3 fatty acid. Many of us fail to get enough fish and vegetables in our diets. Fruits are a little easier to remember to eat. If your diet is lacking any of these foods, make an effort to start including more of them.

We have learned some hints about food preparation that have made the First Place program easy to use. When you buy produce at the store, immediately prepare it for use. How many times have you taken broccoli out of the refrigerator after it has been there a week or so and found it ruined? If you'll chop it up and put it in a food storage bag when you get home, it will be ready to steam or pop into the microwave and fix quick-ly. You will be more likely to use it if it is already prepared.

Many kinds of meat at the grocery store come ready to fix. Chicken breasts can be bought frozen in a bag. Marinate them overnight. You can grill a chicken breast, bake a potato in the microwave and steam mixed vegetables in as short a time as you could cook a frozen dinner. However, it takes planning and a mind-set change.

Many Americans have gravitated to programs that involve a liquid diet. A friend once told me, "You shouldn't give fat people choices." She liked the idea of drinking something five times a day and not needing to choose any foods. People have lost a lot of weight on these programs; however, most people have gained it all back, plus more. These programs cut your calories so low—usually under 500 calories a day—that your body's metabolism also drops to a very slow rate. As soon as you begin eating again, your body is not working as it should, and you put the weight back on faster than you could ever imagine.

Other weight-loss plans provide food with proper nutrition, but you have to buy the food from the distributors. These plans work for a period of time because they provide the right amounts of food. You do not have to make choices. In every one of these plans, a time comes when you have to begin making choices for yourself. Most people do not want to eat preprepared foods indefinitely. They can be expensive and lack variety. If you begin making your own choices again and have not changed your behavior or mind-set, in time you will probably revert to old patterns of eating.

THE BATTLE OF THE MIND

Mind-set change is essential to success in eating right. Most of my problems with eating the wrong foods start in my mind. I must stop the thought process immediately, or usually I'm destined to buy or eat something that I shouldn't.

Years ago a popular ice-cream store carried the food of choice for me. Sometimes I would travel out of my way just to pass by the ice-cream shop. All the time I'd be thinking, *I may not stop there. I may not turn in.* But my mind was already made up. When I drove near the shop, I always turned in and I always bought ice cream.

This situation is very similar to going through the pastry section of the grocery store. We say we're not going to buy anything and then we begin to think, *Well, maybe the kids need something,* or, *Maybe I ought to get something for my husband.* Before we know it, that "something" is in our possession. On the way home, it's in our mouths.

Many times we blame our children for our food choices. We use them as an excuse for having foods in the house that we shouldn't have. I refuse to have anything in my house that can get me in trouble, because I'm not a disciplined person. If I have ice cream in the freezer, I'm the one who is going to eat it. I can say I buy it for the grandchildren, but that's not true. I know when I buy it, I'll be eating it. Therefore, we only have healthy snacks in our house, such as fruit and microwave popcorn. Those are the foods our grandchildren have when they are at our house. They love to eat frozen grapes, watermelon and apples. Our children will eat foods that are healthy if we make those foods available.

We say we can't afford to keep healthy foods in the house because they cost more. However, when we begin to price foods such as potato chips and cookies, we see that we could buy a lot of fruits and vegetables for the same amount of money. We have to get a new mind-set and realize God will help us change our lifestyle if we'll let Him change the way we think.

When the thought of eating something that is not a healthful choice for us enters our minds, we have to stop and pray, *Lord, I'm thinking about this again; help me to think about something else.* Ephesians 2:3 explains this very principle: "All of us also lived among them at one time, gratifying the cravings of our sinful nature." Then verses 8-10 provide the solution to this dilemma:

> For it is by grace that you have been saved, through faith—and this not from yourselves, it is the gift of God—not by works, so that no one can boast. For we are God's workmanship, created in Christ Jesus to do good works, which God prepared in advance for us to do.

The only way that you can change who you are and what you are is to change what goes into your mind. We are products of what we think about. In Philippians 4:8 we are told to fill our minds with "whatever is noble, whatever is right, whatever is pure." This verse also applies to our eating habits. We will eat the kinds of foods we think about.

Denise Castleman of Camden, Arkansas, reminds us of the limitless possibilities available to us when we put Christ in first place and give Him control over every area of our lives. She wrote:

> I just want you to know how thankful I am for First Place. I lost 11½ pounds this time—my goal was 10 pounds. I'm 6 pounds from my overall goal. If you had told me a few years ago when I

weighed 185 pounds that God was going to burden me about leading a Christ-centered health and nutrition program, I would have said you were nuts! Me—of all people—so unhealthy! God has cleansed me through and through. He is worthy of our praise, not because He's done all this, but just because He's my Sovereign God!

God created us for success. He created us to be overcomers. He created us to be victors in this battle we have fought with weight all these years. Only by trusting in Jesus and then clinging to Him every day of our lives are we going to have the strength to win this battle. If your motivation is to serve the Lord as long as you can, as best you can, recall the promise of Philippians 1:6: "He who began a good work in you will carry it on to completion until the day of Christ Jesus."

Note

1. Richard Couey, *Nutrition for God's Temple*, 2nd ed. (Nashville, TN: LifeWay Press, 1994), p. 28.

CHOOSING TO BE ACCOUNTABLE

Commit to the LORD whatever you do, and your plans will succeed.

PROVERBS 16:3

As a member of a First Place group, you are asked to fill out a Commitment Record each day. A Commitment Record (CR) is a food and commitment diary. On the form you record not only what you eat but also how much you eat. Your CR will show you exactly what foods you are lacking and areas where you are overeating. The CR reveals what you are doing and what you are failing to do in all the nine commitment areas. Every good, sound weight-loss program has some method of keeping a record of how you are progressing.

KEEPS US ON TRACK

When I became a leader, I wasn't filling out my CR daily. During the leader's meetings on Wednesday nights, I tried to reconstruct what I had eaten the previous week. I remember Dottie Brewer saying, "It's kind of hard to reconstruct a whole week in five minutes, isn't it, Carole?" I got the point! I have found even today that if I keep a CR, I stay on the Live-It plan. If I don't keep a CR, I have trouble sticking to the plan.

At your weekly group meeting, you will turn in your Commitment Record to your leader. The CR is also a method of communication between you and your leader. We stress accountability, not so your leader can judge and criticize you, but so you can be encouraged to make good choices.

One of our leaders refers to the CR as her best friend. It is a helpful daily reminder in each of the nine commitment areas. So think of your CR as a good friend, not a policeman!

Accountability keeps us on track. Having to write those sugary desserts on our CR keeps us from eating so many of them. Anytime we eat something that is not on the Live-It plan, we still need to record it on the CR. You may have been on diet plans that would require you to skip lunch to stay within your calorie count for the day if you had strayed and eaten a candy bar. In First Place if you eat that candy bar, you still record it on the CR. Then at your next meal, practice good nutrition by eating healthfully. This habit sets your mind on doing the right thing. While you may have gone over in calories for the day, it's not going to make a great difference as long as you don't routinely stray from the plan.

Debbie of Colorado Springs, Colorado, told us,

> Weight had been a problem all of my life and it was getting out of control. I tried to lower my fat content but thought the accountability of a group plus the Bible study might make a difference. Not only did I lose weight, I became a leader of a First Place group. Leadership added a new dimension of accountability. I became excited to lead and learned so much about the process from the members. As I told them, "I'm on the same journey, the same road. I'm just a few weeks ahead of you. Let's walk forward together. It's an exciting journey."

REVEALS TRENDS

We can hide so much from ourselves. We may be eating larger amounts than we need. When we measure and weigh our food portions, the truth is revealed to us. John 8:32 tells us, "The truth will set you free." John was not speaking concerning food in this passage, but the truth about what we eat, how much we eat and why we eat can free us from the bondage of food.

Your body needs approximately 45 different nutrients daily. Fourteen hundred calories is the minimum you can eat to get these essential nutrients. If you don't eat all of the foods that are indicated on the exchange list, you're going to be lacking in some of the vitamins and minerals you need for that day. Some of these the body does not store, making our daily food intake vitally important to good health.

Omitting foods from any category turns First Place into another fad diet. You need a variety of foods on your CR. The beauty of the exchange program is you will find food in each group on the exchange list that you do like to eat. We don't want you to feel obligated to eat foods you don't like. We teach you to go through the exchange list and highlight the foods you like to eat. You will see how broad your choices are—or how limited.

Then you can try adding some of the foods you didn't originally highlight. Many have discovered new food choices that they truly enjoy. Asparagus, not a popular choice for everyone, was found to be high on the list of one member after his wife prepared an asparagus casserole. Other not-so-popular foods have become edible choices for many of us as we learn how fruits, meats, grains and vegetables have their own distinct tastes. Many of us have eaten foods covered with butter, cheese or cream sauce for so long that we think everything should taste that way. You will enjoy the new tastes you discover.

In addition to your food choices, you will record on your CR the amount of water you drink. Your body needs at least 64 ounces of water every day: this amount is the equivalent of eight eight-ounce glasses. You may be among the many who are not water drinkers. Some of us have used colas, fruit juice, tea and other beverages to quench our thirst. Drinking an adequate amount of water and having good health, however, seem to have a correlation. Knowing the need for water and the effects of not having enough water can help us form the habit of drinking more water daily. Once our bodies are used to consuming more water, we will have the desire for it.

REINFORCES OTHER COMMITMENTS

As important as the nutritional part of the CR is, the places for recording the other commitments are every bit as important. The CR has a place for you to check when you've read your Scripture, had your prayer time and encouraged another class member for the week. The CR also asks what exercise you did and how long you did it. This ongoing record reflects the extent to which you are keeping the commitments you have made. The commitments other than the Live-It plan are even more important than the foods you eat. If you keep these commitments, eventually your food choices will fall into line. As a result, you can get stronger and become more committed to what you are doing.

Sometimes you may fail to start your CR on the first day of the week or you may skip a day or more. You may even find yourself skipping a week! If you don't fill out a CR, we ask you to put your name on one and write a note to your leader explaining why you didn't fill it out that week. Your leader will want to know why you're not doing one of the commitments so he or she can pray for you. Whether you have a reason or an excuse, you need to have somebody in your group pray with you about it, so the next week may flow more smoothly. Sometimes there are good reasons for not doing a CR for the week. Remember, we are not looking for perfect people in First Place, just committed people.

Your CR is a convenient size to fold and keep in your billfold or purse if you work outside the home. If you are at home most of the time, you might want to keep it on your refrigerator, so you see it frequently. The CR is yours and is meant to help you. Discover what works best for you.

After you reach your goal, you don't have to fill out a Commitment Record. However, most of my leaders who are at their goal weight still fill out a CR every week. Most people find filling out a CR is helpful in maintaining their goals. It guides them in making correct choices in all food groups. When you increase your calorie intake after you reach your goal, you will find the CR to be a regular reminder of what led to your attaining your goal. The bottom line is that when we are accountable, we have a much better chance of maintaining our weight goals once we reach them.

And for those of you who are new to First Place, the CR is going to be one of the most important commitments you will make in the program. It will change your life.

Choosing to Exercise

Do you not know that in a race all the runners run, but only one gets the prize? Run in such a way as to get the prize. Everyone who competes in the games goes into strict training. They do it to get a crown that will not last; but we do it to get a crown that will last forever. Therefore I do not run like a man running aimlessly; I do not fight like a man beating the air. No, I beat my body and make it my slave so that after I have preached to others, I myself will not be disqualified for the prize.

1 Corinthians 9:24-27

Exercise is the ninth and final commitment of the First Place program. This commitment is definitely one of those that we must deliberately choose to do. Personally, it is one of my favorites, because exercising on a regular basis has been life changing for me. After I started my running program in January of 1985, God began to teach me that if an undisciplined person like me would exercise on a regular basis, He would use that discipline in other areas of my life. He would make changes in other areas of my life as I yielded to His Lordship.

DEVELOPING THE HABIT

I can't say there are a lot of things about exercise that I like. First of all, I don't like to sweat. And I sweat when I exercise. I don't like to wash my hair every day, but I have to when I exercise at an aerobic level. Many times, I just don't feel like exercising when I get up in the mornings. Sometimes I just wake up in a bad mood, for whatever reason, and don't want to exercise. I want to stay in bed, drink coffee at home and read the newspaper.

Exercise also requires self-discipline—something I usually resist. Writing this book has been a difficult process for me because I don't like to do anything requiring discipline. You might look at my life and think I am a disciplined person, but I'm really not. I'm lazy in many areas and I don't want to be disciplined.

But I do enjoy some aspects of exercise. I love the way it makes me feel after I finish a workout. Plus when I'm having a bad day, I remember that only 5 percent of the people in the world exercise on a regular basis. Just think, I'm in that 5 percent and you can be, too. If you suffer from low self-esteem, exercising on a regular basis can help turn that around. You have made a commitment to do something that most of the world does not do.

Exercise has also given me a sense of organization. I tried time-management classes to help me with my lack of organization. I attended these classes and thought they were wonderful. In fact, I attended four different times! And I bought an organizer to get more organized. I now own three or four; however, they are unused. Instead, God has organized my entire life through my commitment to exercise.

When I exercise, I am able to plan my day. It's a time for me to think about the coming day's events. I can pray about what I know is on my agenda, and I can pray for guidance on how to handle the unexpected events that will occur. I can ask God to give me the strength to be Christlike in every dealing I have that day. I can ask Him to help me treat everybody I meet the way God would want me to treat them.

I was not always at this place in my life. Getting into an exercise routine was not an easy task for me—but I had to start somewhere.

In First Place we give you that place to start: We ask you to commit to exercise three times a week. This much aerobic exercise is necessary for a person to stay physically fit. Those who are just beginning an exercise program need to commit to building up to exercise five times a week. Regular exercise is essential to the First Place program, as attested to by Kathy Smith of Omaha, Nebraska. She wrote,

The only way I found I could continue to maintain consistent weight loss was through exercise. I decided to exercise every day as much as possible. I did not want to battle every day with "should I or shouldn't I," so I just decided to make it a part of every day. I don't have to battle excuses like "I'm too tired today" or "It's too cold." (It does get REAL cold in Nebraska!) It turned out to be a very good decision.

Dr. Dick Couey is a well-known Christian motivational speaker on the subject of physical fitness. After one of his speeches, an elderly lady approached him and said, "I don't know how I can exercise. I can just barely walk." Dick replied, "Then you just barely walk." That's what she started doing. I've read stories of 90-year-old men who could barely walk when they went to a fitness center. They began to walk around a track, and after a few months they were walking three to five miles a day. Their health had returned. Their lifestyle had dramatically changed.

Our bodies will respond if given the proper nutrition and the proper exercise—they will begin to heal themselves. We have seen it happen over and over. We know of women who walked with a cane and now walk perfectly fine without one.

Dear friends, the time to get physically fit is not when you are sick. It's too late to get fit when you are sick. You need to get fit when you are well, even if you are not as well as you would like to be. Even if you think, *I'm not well enough to exercise*, you must start where you are right now. You can start by walking a short distance every day. God will begin to strengthen your body.

FINDING A WORKOUT SCHEDULE

Since I am an undisciplined person, I commit to exercising five times a week. If you're an undisciplined person and you commit to exercise three times a week—Monday, Wednesday and Friday—what happens when you miss Wednesday? The natural tendency of the undisciplined person is to think, *Well, I'll just go ahead and miss Friday, too. I've already missed one time this week—I'll start again next Monday.*

A disciplined person would think, *Well, I missed Wednesday, so I'll do it Thursday and Friday*. Most of us may not think that way. My commitment is to exercise five times a week. If I miss one day, then I'll still be exercising four times a week and maintaining my fitness. If I miss two days, then I still have three days of exercise for that week. In other words, I have a built-in cushion when circumstances change and I can't keep my exercise schedule.

Some things you have to do whether you feel like doing it or not. Many times, I don't feel like getting up and exercising. But I've made that commitment to exercise. Therefore, I put on my clothes and go anyway. I get up at 5:00 A.M. and have my quiet time from 5:00 to 6:00 A.M. I then go and exercise with friends from 6:00 to 7:00 A.M. Morning is the best time for me to exercise, because no one needs me to do anything else that early in the morning.

But you may not be a morning person. I have a friend who is a night person and she decided to start exercising in the mornings. At the first of the year, she said, "I've made a New Year's resolution."

"What's that?" I asked.

"Well, I have resolved to start going to bed earlier, so I can get up and exercise with you at 6:00 A.M."

I replied, "Why not reverse your goal? The goal would be to get up in time to exercise at 6:00 A.M. Then your exercise program is not depending on when you go to bed. You will go to bed earlier as a consequence of getting up earlier. If you get up early three or four weeks in a row and you're exercising at 6:00 A.M., you'll have to start going to bed earlier." Going to bed earlier so that we'll get up earlier hardly ever works, so make early rising your goal.

Many people exercise after work. If you will make the commitment to do so, exercising in the early evening will work well. Most high schools have a quarter-mile track where you may walk every day.

It's also helpful to have a friend to exercise with. However, some of the people I see walking together in my neighborhood are not walking at an aerobic rate. I would recommend getting an audiocassette player and listening to Scripture cassettes/CDs or ones specifically designed to keep you at an aerobic pace. But be careful: Don't let headphones distract you from traffic and other hazards!

Perhaps you're thinking, *Well, I can't exercise because I have a preschooler at home.* But many of our young mothers use aerobic cassettes at home, and their preschoolers love doing the exercises with them. Aerobic cassettes for children are available, and parents can use these and benefit from them as well.

I myself have taken my granddaughter Cara with me to exercise since she was very small. We went to the track at the high school when she was about four years old. As I jogged, she rode beside me on her bike with training wheels. When she grew older, she loved to come to the church and jog in the mornings. Learn to see exercise as a way to spend quality time with your children that benefits you physically as well.

Children and spouses are not a hindrance to our exercising. We are the hindrance. We say we can't do it. The best thing we could ever do for our family members is to spend time with them. Walking or jogging is a good time for meaningful conversation with children or a spouse. Several generations ago much talking and teaching were done as family members shared farm tasks. Grandmothers, mothers and daughters spent time together sewing and canning. Although lifestyles have changed, we must find times when we can do things together. What better activity to share than exercise! And what better way to help our children and other family members learn healthy living!

ENJOYING THE BENEFITS

Exercise has been a special spiritual blessing to me. My exercise time has allowed me to see how faithful the Lord is and how He has answered my prayers, helping me keep my First Place commitments.

Many times, I have talked to the Lord on the way to the church and told Him that I'm going to exercise. I remind Him that 80 percent of life is showing up, and therefore, I'm showing up. But I tell myself that I'm not going to exercise very much that day—I'm only going to jog a mile. Every time I've said that, God has blessed me with a friend showing up to run with me—someone with whom I don't normally exercise, who will exercise with me and encourage me. For a while, a friend ran with me who also had his quiet time before jogging. He would share with me what he had studied in his Bible. I was blessed not only to get in my exercise but also to learn from a fellow Christian.

Your exercise time is a wonderful opportunity to enrich your mind as well as your body. I listen to our Scripture verses put to music while I exercise. But I have also listened to sermons and motivational audiocassettes. In fact, when I first began exercising in 1985, a friend gave me a grocery bag full of cassettes. In the bag was a series of cassettes by Zig Ziglar with motivational music that went along with his book *See You at the Top*. Each morning for six weeks I listened to the music as I jogged. I would be so pumped up by the time I got to the office that the girls in the office would say, "Would you shut up!" They came in rubbing their eyes and trying to get awake, while I had been motivated for an hour to think about the things that are really important in life. I had been thinking about goals, achievement, people and the ones that I love. I was motivated to start the day.

My mother is in her 80s, and she is such an example to me of the importance of keeping physically fit. Even though she can't now, for years she walked three miles a day. She was fit and healthy. Yet I don't think I appreciated the value of her walking routine until six years ago, when we were on a vacation in Galveston, Texas. We had rented a beach house for the week. My mother became ill while we were there, and within about an hour, she had 103° fever. We decided to take her to the hospital, and we had to ride a ferry across to Galveston to the hospital. In a matter of a very few hours, her fever was 105°. She spent most of the night in the waiting room in a wheelchair because it was a holiday weekend and the hospital was very busy. After she was finally put in a room, they diagnosed her illness as streptococcal septicemia, a deadly strep infection of the blood. This is the same illness that struck Jim Henson, creator of the Muppets on *Sesame Street*, killing him within a very few hours.

But the outcome of the story is that she did not die from the raging infection that attacked her body. One of the doctors told me if she had not been a walker, her heart would not have been strong enough to withstand the strep infection.

Today my mother can no longer walk for exercise, because she has arthritis. She does water aerobics with a group of senior adults. In the summer, they exercise at the pool in their apartment complex. During the winter, they use an indoor heated pool.

The lesson for us is that the time never comes when we can't exercise, if we really want to. Sometimes exercise is a little inconvenient for us, but it will pay great dividends if we'll make the time to keep this commitment.

USING AN EXERCISE LOG

When I began walking, I kept a personal log of when and how much I exercised. The use of a log to record my progress has not only encouraged and inspired me but also has served as a record of steady progress toward my own personal fitness goals.

In the First Place program we ask that you, too, keep an exercise log. This log is a simple weekly record of the dates, distance and duration of each workout, as well as the type of exercise (walking, running, swimming, etc.). We also encourage you to record in your log your thoughts for each day.

If you miss a week, that's okay. But be sure to write across that page what was going on that week and why you couldn't exercise. Just as with the CR, remember that we are looking for committed people, not perfect ones.

I still keep a weekly exercise log—and I still occasionally miss my workout. My overall goal, however, is still to never exercise less than I did the year before. This should be your goal as well. See your exercise log as an essential element of your fitness program—one that will help you achieve a new level of fitness and better health.

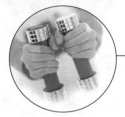

CHAPTER THREE

CHOOSING TO BE A WINNER:
FIRST PLACE VICTORIES

When we reach our weight-loss goals in First Place, we feel tremendous joy in that accomplishment. Success, however, is not found simply in achieving our goals but in the process of change itself. God changes us in the mental, physical, spiritual and emotional areas of our lives. God wants to have a relationship with each one of us that allows Him to be a loving Father who gives good things to each child. Before God can give us the good things He wants for us, many areas of our lives must be healed.

In this chapter I would like to share with you stories of First Place victories. Each story you read will tell you how God has radically changed these individuals through their involvement in the First Place program. But they are quick to point out that it was not the program itself but the relationship with our heavenly Father that caused the changes.

These testimonies are meant to encourage you. They were written by people just like you—people who made a decision to put Christ first. It is my hope that as they tell their stories, they will speak to you. I pray that you, too, will be inspired to choose to change.

KAREN ARNETT
EVANS, GEORGIA

When I was four years old, I went to live with my grandparents for a few months. When my parents came to get me, they hardly recognized me. My grandmother had fed me very well.

Although I was a very active child, I remained overweight. Looking back, I know I mostly overate from boredom. Diets wouldn't work because I used food to keep me busy, to comfort me and to push down any anxiety that I had.

It wasn't until I found First Place that I came to realize that only God could truly help me. Only by committing all of my life to Him and disciplining myself could I overcome my eating problem. With the help and support of people who cared, I was able to commit myself whole-heartedly to God and follow the First Place program.

God has blessed me in all areas of my life since then. I have lost 245 pounds and 83½ inches. I have gone from a size 56 to a 10 or 12. I have been able to maintain for three months now. At one time I had great difficulty just standing in the back of a room and talking. Now I am a First Place leader and I give my testimony at local churches. It is amazing what God has done in my life.

When I was overweight, I was not a testimony to who God was and to the power He had in my life. I didn't use the power He had given me. But now God has used the weakest area of my life to exhibit His power.

I would like to remind all of you that each part of the First Place program is important. If we will keep all of our commitments, First Place works. Each commitment builds on the others. Each commitment supports the others. Don't take your commitments lightly. You aren't committing to your leader, your spouse or your friend; you are committing to God. God is faithful. He never breaks a promise. Each of the promises in His Word is a commitment to us. He is calling us to faithfulness. When you make a commitment, you are making a promise to be faithful.

KATHIE SMITH
DAVIE, FLORIDA

Before I came to First Place, my life was a blur of doing everything but not doing anything very well. I worked as a carrier for the U.S. Postal Service for 10 years while trying to be a good wife and mother and still find time to devote to God and my church. I kept up a good front, but in reality things were slipping out of control. I had turned 40 in November, but even before that I was fighting a losing battle with my weight, and I was tired all the time.

My husband and I had prayed for several years that I could quit my job and find something to do part-time, so I could be here for our children. Yet every idea we came up with hit a dead end, until God finally showed us how we could make it on one income. So I retired from the post office on Christmas Eve, and I thanked God for answering my long-time prayer request. I prayed that I would find a ministry that would fill the free time I had while my children were in school but still leave me with flexibility, so I could be there when they needed me. And I also wanted to get in shape. So right after the first of the year I began walking in the morning after I dropped the kids off at school. But something was missing. I needed more than exercise—I needed accountability.

I had heard of First Place from a few area churches and was interested, but I just didn't want to go to another church. I had begun walking once a week with my pastor's wife, Pam McCord, and mentioned this to her. She said she would also like to attend but wished the First Place program would come to our church one day. After much prayer, God led me to my friend, Mary Ann Rowe, who had worked in the field of fitness and nutrition for 15 years. As a result, First Place was brought to First Baptist Church of West Hollywood, Florida. After months of preparation, we began our first class with 13 women.

I am now leading a First Place group at my church. And I am just as excited as I was when I started in 1997. I can't tell enough people what a wonderful program First Place is. It changes lives. Most people tell me they joined the group to lose weight, but what they have gained is a closer relationship with the Lord. What a blessing!

PAULA V. STACEY
MONROEVILLE, ALABAMA

I can't believe that I am writing this testimony, but it is due to God's empowerment and loving care. In May 1995, I began First Place in

Monroeville. Was I apprehensive! I was scared, but I had reached the point that I was ready to do something about my weight. The first time I stepped on the scales, I weighed 295 pounds, wore a size 26 and was in terrible health.

I began the program and did it by the books—*First Place* and the Bible! After the first week, I stepped on the scales and I hadn't lost an ounce. I fell to pieces. But I persevered and soon began losing consistently. As I write this testimony, I have lost 140 pounds and I wear a size 10 or 12. I have lost over 100 inches over the past 21 months. More important, I have grown so much spiritually. I have allowed God to empower me to control my eating and exercise habits. He has taught me discipline in so many areas of my life. I am a changed person on the outside and inside. I am so grateful for God's provision of this program.

I encourage you to work the First Place program, just as it is written. The success of the program lies in the nine commitments you make. Each commitment is so important, but I have to mention two of my favorites.

First, the one that has meant the most to me is the memorizing of Scripture. I remember thinking, *How can memorizing Scripture help me lose weight? That's ridiculous!* But it did. It gave me encouragement and the ability to stay focused on the enormous task that lay ahead. The Scriptures taught me that I can't, but God can (see Phil. 4:13).

Second, as a former couch potato, I can honestly say that I have really grown to love exercising. I can see and feel its benefits. I have learned that it releases stress and makes you feel good about yourself. It has become a natural part of my life—just like breathing. It's something I enjoy doing. It is a huge factor in my success in First Place.

I give praise to God for the staff of First Place (past and present) and their heeding of God's leading. I also thank God for my family, my friends in First Place and my church family, all of whom encouraged me as I strove toward the goal. You'll never know how much the calls, cards and comments helped me stay the course—and still do! Lastly and most important, I praise God for His intervention in my life through First Place. I worked hard, prayed hard and gave it to God, and God worked a miracle! He can do it for you too—if you give Him first place!

SHEILA ROBBINS
HOUSTON, TEXAS

I had always been an overweight teenager and adult. I tried every new fad diet that came along, including diet pills, the liquid protein diet, the low-carbohydrate diet and the grapefruit diet. And sometimes I even did the starvation routine. By 1981, I weighed 295 pounds. The new weight-loss craze on the agenda was to have my stomach stapled. Six long months after surgery, I had lost 60 pounds. But by 1983, I had stretched out my stomach, and I was back to my old eating habits. My weight was on its way back up again.

In September 1985, a very special lady from my church introduced the First Place program to a small group of women. Now weighing 320 pounds, I was very reluctant to attend the orientation because of my numerous weight-loss failures. But with her encouragement, I attended. At the end of the First Place orientation, the group had a special prayer for commitment. During the prayer time, the Holy Spirit spoke to me. I realized that I had allowed this weight problem to remain *my problem*, and I had never given it to the Lord. God began to impress on me that my body is the dwelling place of His gracious Spirit. On that day, my life changed in way that I had never imagined it could.

By 1987, I had lost around 150 pounds. But the weight loss was only the beginning of what God had in store for me.

I cared so deeply for First Place attendees like myself, who thought because they were obese, they were unlovable and life was barely worth living. As my weight began coming off, people began to notice my outward appearance. I found that I could use their attention to my weight loss as an opportunity to tell them that there is hope in a seemingly hopeless situation. I became a First Place leader and began to share with them not only about the food and exercise program but also about First Place's emphasis on prayer and Bible study. I found myself witnessing about Christ to people—good friends, total strangers, anyone who had been watching me shrink to half my former size. Before my weight loss, I doubt that I would have witnessed about Christ.

Today, maintaining my weight can still be a struggle. Yet I know that God's grace is sufficient. I have victory over my weight as I continue to put Christ first in my life. Thank you, Jesus, for the First Place program and for those who step out every day to give you first place!

MARTHA ROGERS
HOUSTON, TEXAS

When our youngest son and his new bride brought over their wedding album for us to see, I realized for the first time that I had lost control of my weight. For many years our church had sponsored a First Place program, but I didn't want to bother with a regimented program. After weeks of trying to lose with my own plan and not having any success, I decided I needed help. I talked with Carole Lewis, the First Place director, and she convinced me that First Place was where I needed to be. I joined in March and by November had lost 44 pounds and reached my goal weight. The regular exercise and healthy eating gave me energy and a new outlook on life. In addition, the Bible study, Scripture reading and memory verses strengthened my relationship with God. I became a leader of a group and shared how God had blessed me through First Place.

I had no idea God was preparing me for the greatest test of faith and courage I had ever encountered. A little less than a year after I reached my goal, a biopsy revealed a malignant tumor in my breast. Fear, anxiety, despair and helplessness took over my every thought for the first few days after the diagnosis. As I prepared for surgery, I began to think of the Bible verses I had memorized in First Place. Jeremiah 29:11 "'For I know the plans I have for you,' declares the LORD, 'plans to prosper you and not to harm you, plans to give you hope and a future'"; and Philippians 4:19: "My God will meet all your needs according to his glorious riches in Christ Jesus." My fears and anxiety went away. I knew God would take care of me in any and all circumstances.

After the surgery, the doctors decided no chemo or radiation treatments would be needed. In addition, because of my body's healthy condition, my recovery took less time than usual. My surgeon and oncologist were quick to credit my good health as the main contributing factor in my recovery. My regular doctor, a Christian, also credits my great faith in God's promises.

Within a few weeks I had recovered completely and was able to return to my teaching job. At the end of the first month, I had resumed my full slate of activities, including leading my First Place class. I know the First Place program provided not only for my physical needs through a healthy body, but it also took care of my spiritual needs through the verses I had memorized.

Nothing else can give you a healthy body, mind, spirit and soul like First Place. Through the Bible studies I have a much closer relationship with God. I no longer worry about what happens in my life, because I know who is in control. Together, good health and a mind focused on Christ carried me through what could have been a dark time in my life, to become a shining example of God's love and mercy.

LYNNE RUSSELL
DEER PARK, TEXAS

In April 1996, I found myself to be in a severely depleted condition. Physically, I was experiencing muscle and joint pain, fatigue, high cholesterol and high blood pressure. Emotionally, I was worn and frustrated. There seemed to be no way out of the struggle over medical treatments, weekly doctor visits and lack of energy for the activities necessary for work, church and family. The physical fatigue was also affecting my ability to function mentally. I felt tired and dull, especially spiritually.

The doctor recommend I consult with a rheumatologist for more aggressive treatment (chemotherapy) for lupus, which caused my muscle and joint pain, weakness and fatigue. The mental and emotional sluggishness seemed to be related as well. At the same time, the doctor gave me an article about fibromyalgia (muscle pain) and walking. I cried. I couldn't walk; it hurt too much. Nobody understood. I left the doctor's office that day, aggravated and a little afraid. I knew that anything else the doctors had to offer would only rob me of the little energy I had left. I had nowhere to look but up.

I began to ask for wisdom and help. As always, when I ask, God responds. I was convicted to make an effort to walk and to trust God with my overall health. I cancelled the appointment with the rheumatologist and joined a new Sunday morning First Place group in our church. I work evenings, but God still provided a class that I could attend. My first week I progressed from walking five minutes in agony to walking 15 minutes without much difficulty. Within three weeks I was walking a 20-minute mile, eating healthier and participating in daily Bible study.

In January 1997, I returned to the doctor's office for lab work and found that my cholesterol level had dropped, and the ANA count (lupus factor) was below normal, with no treatments needed for six months. It has been years now since I began this physical, spiritual, emotional and mental journey. God has blessed me with a 55-pound weight loss and freedom from pain, fatigue and high cholesterol levels. I now gladly share what He has done in my life through First Place to give testimony to His love and great power.

KAY SMITH
FIRST PLACE ASSOCIATE DIRECTOR
HOUSTON, TEXAS

I grew up in the country and being overweight did not seem like much of a problem until I reached my teenage years. I told our family physician I wanted to lose weight. He prescribed diet pills and told me to take the pills and stop eating. I did, and it worked. But I found that I would also gain weight back very fast when I stopped the pills and went back to eating what I wanted. I began this yo-yo pattern at a very early age and continued it for more than 25 years.

My husband and I spent thousands of dollars on every weight-loss gimmick that became available. My own personal physician tried to help by having me weigh in each week. The office visit was free if I lost weight, and I paid double if I gained.

My family fully supported every attempt I made, and I can tell you that they suffered. The emotional highs and lows of someone addicted to diet pills are not unlike any other chemical addiction. When I committed to never take diet pills again, it was a wise decision, but the weight went up, up, up. My health began to suffer. I could barely walk. I suffered tremendous foot problems and was told if I didn't lose weight, I would end up in a wheelchair. I did not fit in a chair at the movies and would not even think of an airplane trip, knowing the seat belt would not fasten. I remember the fear I felt when my Sunday School class discussed a backyard party. I knew a lawn chair was an impossibility and sitting on the ground required several people to help me up. I was never honest with anyone about these thoughts, except my husband. I exhibited a happy-go-lucky nature that hid my inner pain.

I remember so well the Monday that I sat down in the empty sanctuary at my church and told God that I didn't want to live anymore. I felt completely helpless to overcome this tremendous problem in my life. I had truly hit bottom. That day I told God, "I give up. I am unable to control this area of my life." I believe that time alone in the sanctuary was one of the spiritual markers in my life. I was so aware of God's presence and of His assurance that this was not too big of a problem for Him. I went into the church office and spoke to a good friend. I was honest with her about my depression and I asked her if she had ever heard of any Christian weight-loss programs. She got me in touch with First Place.

Reluctantly, I attended the orientation. I listened as each commitment was explained and thought, *I think I could do that.* It was not a surprise to me to realize that I needed some discipline in my life. I felt such assurance that this was where God wanted me; and the more I heard about the program, I believed that God had made it just for me. I did not lose a single pound at that orientation, but I felt like I had lost 100 pounds. I did not understand how God was going to do this, but I believed He could. I had been given hope.

It has not been an easy journey. The weight loss of 90 pounds has been fantastic, but it doesn't compare to the other blessings I have received.

I never dreamed that I needed any emotional healing. I learned how much better relationships can be when you learn how to share emotional pain and joy.

First Place also taught me how to have a personal daily relationship with Jesus. God's Word and the personal time spent with Him have given me the strength I need each day. One of the greatest blessings in my life is that the fear of gaining this weight back is gone—because of Him.

While I have truly made a permanent lifestyle change and I consider it my privilege to eat healthy and exercise, I also realize that you cannot fail First Place. I believe that the success is in the process.

And while I do not believe God caused me to be overweight, He did take this weakness in my life and use it to draw me into a relationship with Him—a relationship that is molding me into a servant He can use. One of my life verses is Philippians 1:6: "Being confident of this, that he who began a good work in you will carry it on to completion until the day of Christ Jesus." Hear the promise, as I did, and believe that it is meant for you, too!

CHAPTER FOUR

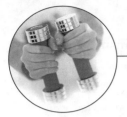

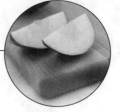

CHOOSING CHRIST

The most important choice you will ever make is the decision to put Christ first in your life. If you have not already made that commitment, prayerfully read the following verses that explain how to become a Christian.

BECOMING A CHRISTIAN

God loves you and has a wonderful plan for your life.

> *For God so loved the world that He gave his one and only Son,*
> *that whoever believes in him shall not perish but*
> *have eternal life.*
> —John 3:16

Many people feel life is not so wonderful and that is because man is sinful and is separated from God who is perfect.

> *All have sinned and fall short of the glory of God.*
> —Romans 3:23

God created man for fellowship with Him, but man chose his own way and separated himself from God. I am a sinner. Are you?

> *The wages of sin is death, but the gift of God is eternal life in*
> *Christ Jesus our Lord.*
> —Romans 6:23

Even though the only payment for our sins is death, many people try to get close to God by doing good works and going to church. But Jesus said,

I am the way and the truth and the life. No one comes to
the Father except through me.
—John 14:6

The only way to God is through His Son, Jesus Christ, who died on the cross for you and for me.

For it is by grace you have been saved, through faith—and this not from
yourselves, it is the gift of God—not by works, so that no one can boast.
—Ephesians 2:8,9

God gives you Himself as a free gift. But a gift must be accepted.

Everyone who calls on the name of the Lord will be saved.
—Romans 10:13

Are you willing to turn from your sins and to Jesus? If so, pray this prayer:

Jesus, thank You for loving me and dying on the cross for me. Please for-
give me of my sins and help me to give my life totally to You. Come into
my life and be my Lord and Savior. Amen.

STEPS FOR SPIRITUAL GROWTH

- Prayer offers opportunity to praise and thank God and receive guidance.
- Reading the Bible keeps us grounded in God's Word for daily living.

- Our local church provides fellowship with other believers and a place of worship.
- Service through the local church is an expression of our gratitude and faith.
- Witnessing is our opportunity to share the good news with others.

And remember, faith is a gift that grows as we use it!

ABOUT THE AUTHOR

Carole Lewis is the national director of First Place:
A Christ-Centered Health Program, which originated
in 1981 at Houston's First Baptist Church. Carole was
a member of the original First Place group and
became the full-time director of the program in 1987.
Carole has seen the program grow from 12 people in
one church to thousands of members in 12,000
churches, representing every state and many
foreign counties.

Carole is married to Johnny, and they have three
grown children and eight grandchildren. She has
a deep love of people, and her heart's desire is to see
them become what God created them to be. Carole
shares her words of encouragement and motivation
at conferences and seminars across the nation.

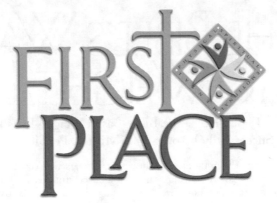

First Place was founded under the providence of God and with the conviction that there is a need for a program which will train the minds, develop the moral character and enrich the spiritual lives of all those who may come within the sphere of its influence.

First Place is dedicated to providing quality information for development of a physical, emotional and spiritual environment leading to a life that honors God in Jesus Christ. As a health-oriented program, First Place will stress the highest excellence and proficiency in instruction with a goal of developing within each participant mastery of all the basics of a lasting healthy lifestyle, so that all may achieve their highest potential in body, mind and spirit. The spiritual development of each participant shall be given high priority so that each may come to the knowledge of Jesus Christ and God's plan and purpose for each life.

First Place offers instruction, encouragement and support to help members experience a more abundant life. Please contact the First Place national office in Houston, Texas at (800) 727-5223 for information on the following resources:

- ❖ Training Opportunities
- ❖ Conferences/Rallies
- ❖ Workshops
- ❖ Fitness Weeks

Send personal testimonies to:

First Place
7401 Katy Freeway
Houston, TX 77024

Phone: **(800) 727-52223**
Website: ***www.firstplace.org***

THE BIBLE'S WAY TO WEIGHT LOSS

First Place—the Bible-Based Weight-Loss Program
Used Successfully by over 1/2 Million People!

Are you one of the millions of disheartened dieters who've tried one fad diet after another without success? If so, your search for a successful diet is over! First Place is the proven weight loss program born over 20 years ago in the First Baptist Church of Houston.

But First Place does much more than help you take off weight and keep it off. This Bible-based program will transform your life in every way—physically, mentally, spiritually and emotionally. Now's the time to join!

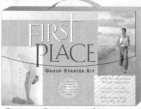

Group Starter Kit
ISBN 08307.28708

Every leader needs a First Place Group Starter Kit. This kit has everything group leaders need to help others change their lives forever by giving God first place! Kits include:

- *Leader's Guide*
- *Member's Guide*
- *Giving Christ First Place Bible Study* with Scripture Memory CD
- *Choosing to Change* by Carole Lewis
- *First Place* by Carole Lewis with Terry Whalin
- *Orientation* Video
- *Nine Commitments* Video
- *Food Exchange Plan* Video

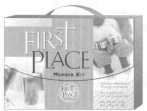

Member Kit
ISBN 08307.28694

Each member needs a First Place Group Starter Kit. All the material is easy to understand and spells out principles members can easily apply in their daily lives. Kit includes:

- *Member's Guide*
- *Choosing to Change* by Carole Lewis
- 13 Commitment Records
- Four Motivational Audiocassettes
- *Prayer Journal*
- Scripture Memory Verses: *Walking in the Word*

ESSENTIAL FIRST PLACE PROGRAM MATERIALS

Giving Christ First Place Bible Study
with Scripture Memory CD
ISBN 08307.28643

Everyday Victory for Everyday People Bible Study
with Scripture Memory CD
ISBN 08307.28651

Available at your local Christian bookstore or by calling **1-800-4-GOSPEL**.

To see other First Place resources, visit **www.gospellight.com/firstplace**.

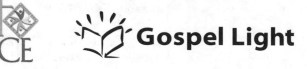